HEALING WISDOM

OF

NORTH AMERICAN

TREES

FROM ROOT TO REMEDY

A Practitioner's Guide to Identification, Traditional Use and Herbal Alchemy

BRENDA GALLAGHER

Cataloguing data available from Library and Archives Canada

978-0-88839-798-0 [paperback]

978-0-88839-799-7 [epub]

Printed in South Korea

Cover Design:	J. Rade
Editor:	D. Martens
Design & Layout:	J. Rade

Publisher's Note
The information in this book is offered for general educational and historical purposes only and is not intended as medical advice. Readers should consult a qualified healthcare professional before using any plant, preparation, or remedy, particularly if pregnant, nursing, taking medication, or managing a health condition. Neither the publisher nor the author accepts any liability for loss, injury, or damage resulting from the use or misuse of the information provided; by reading, you assume full responsibility for your choices and their outcomes.

We acknowledge the support of the Government of Canada through the Canada Book Fund and the Canada Council for the Arts, and of the Province of British Columbia through the British Columbia Arts Council and the Book Publishing Tax Credit.

Published simultaneously in Canada and the United States by

HANCOCK HOUSE PUBLISHERS LTD.
19313 Zero Avenue, Surrey, B.C. Canada V3Z 9R9
288 Martin St, Box 10 [Suite 6], Blaine, WA, USA 98230
www.hancockhouse.com | info@hancockhouse.com

Hancock House gratefully acknowledges the Halkomelem Speaking Peoples whose unceded, shared and asserted traditional territories our offices reside upon.

Dedication

This book is dedicated to my father, who encouraged us to always learn more.

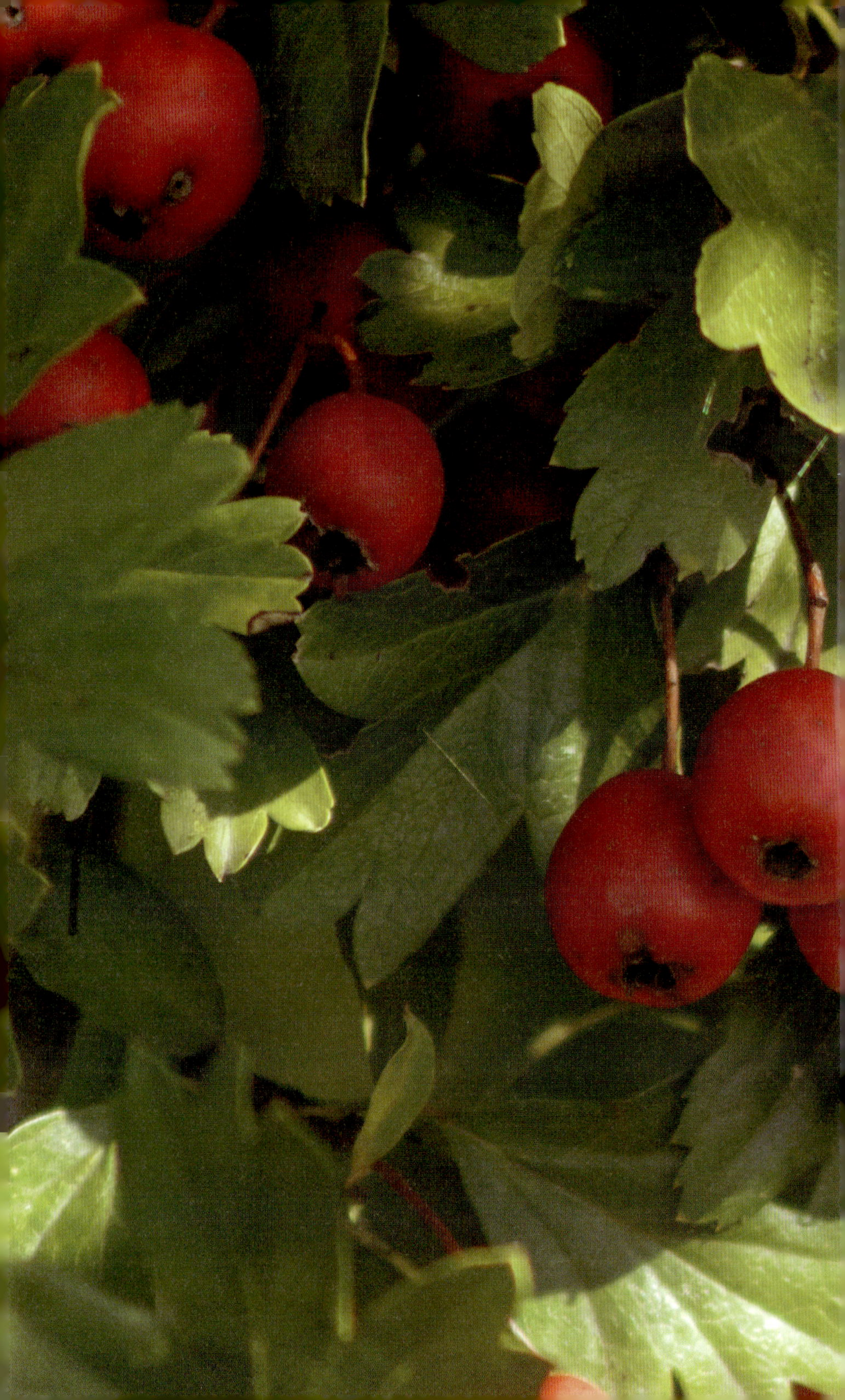

Table of Contents

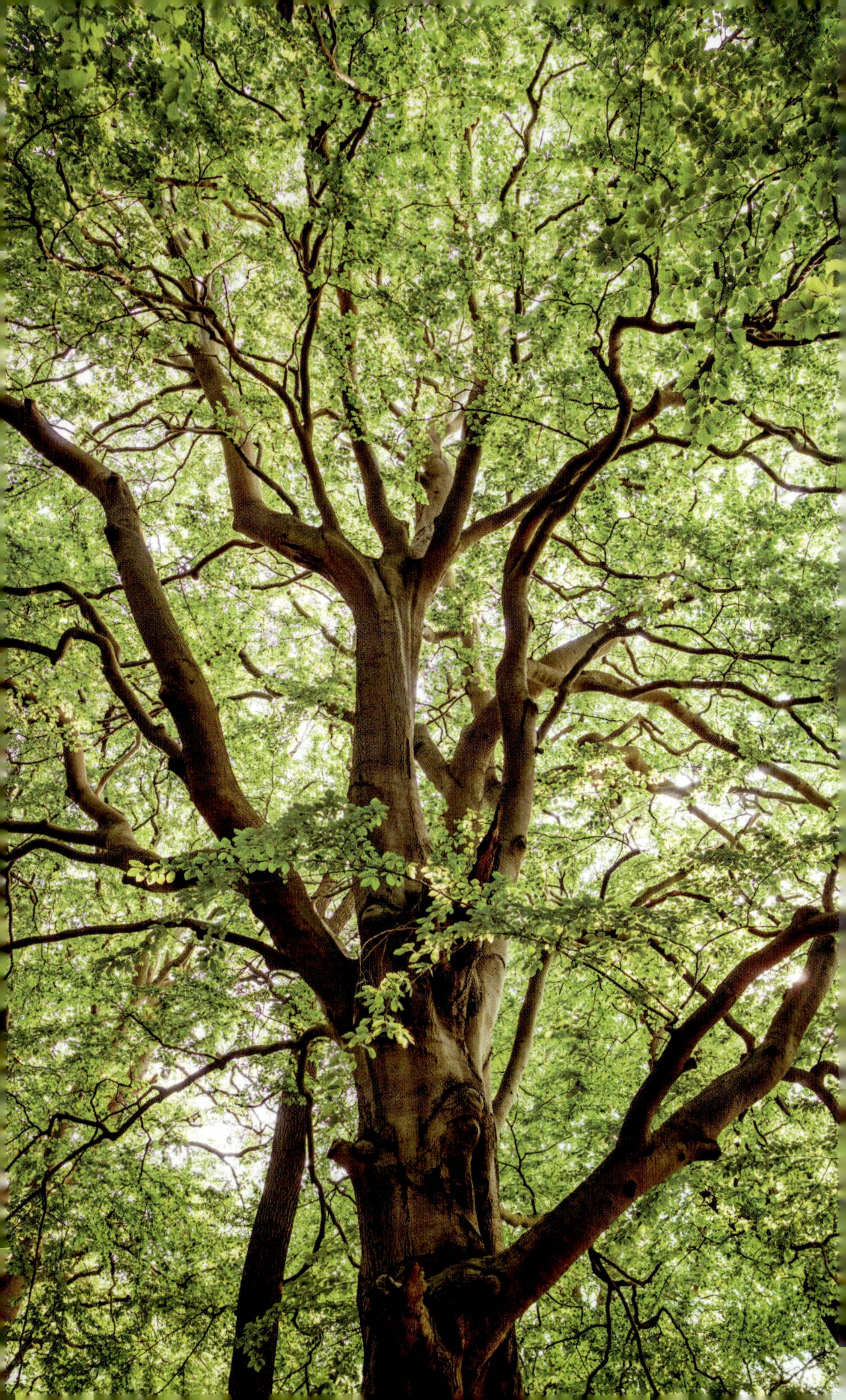

Foreword

A new book about plants is always a welcome addition to the book shelves of those fascinated with plants, though a book about understanding plants, their influence on the environment, their relevance to humans and their rich histories, should be a necessity for all. In our fast-paced world, filled with the stresses of modern society, we often forget about the calming effect of the natural world. Even more so, we forget about our childhood fascination with the non-human entities that surround us everywhere we go. Taking a step back and immersing ourselves into the slow pace of plants can reset our priorities, allowing us to appreciate our origins and understand our place in nature.

The layperson can appreciate the solace provided by a forest, grassland or wetland; a scientist can appreciate the form and function of a healthy ecosystem; a healer can appreciate long-held traditions of gathering plants that have benefited humans for millennia; storytellers can appreciate the human histories tied to our natural world; and all people can appreciate the role plants have played in sustaining ourselves and our families... but rarely does a written work speak to all of these streams of knowledge. Even rarer is finding a practitioner that accepts, understands and can meld these seemingly contradictory approaches to unveil the complexities of nature and the role it plays in our lives. Luckily for us, Brenda Gallagher is such a practitioner.

Educators, naturalists and biologists often strive to translate knowledge of the natural world into a form that others can learn from, borrow from and expand upon. This is no easy task, yet Brenda's written work does so seamlessly and without ego. With a subject matter rooted in complex histories, from western science to oral traditions, from human need to ecological role, this book ties each perspective together in a way that truly increases our understanding of nature and the human connection.

The impact of reading the accounts in this book is akin to joining the author as she travels through rich and biodiverse habitats, as she sits beneath ancient, weathered trees, as she gently harvests fresh leaves, and as she absorbs the energy of nature all around her. At the same time, you unknowingly learn and retain countless minute details about the importance and traditions linked to each plant encountered. Compelling storytelling is a gift few possess, though this book is an exceptional example of how to do it correctly. The author shows her extensive background in understanding western science and how natural communities of wildlife and plants interact with one another, but more than that she reaches beyond academia and science, taking the reader on a journey of discovery, of understanding plant species from various personal and cultural perspectives, seamlessly assimilating information into an accessible and inviting form. The author understands people, she understands natural environments and through decades of experience, she understands that there is no single way to appreciate and embrace the life that surround us.

Providing both a sense of place and purpose, this book traverses boundaries of understanding plants for their medicinal, edible and spiritual potential, of their historical and present significance, of their use for humans and their importance apart from humans. It should come as no surprise that we need to slow our lives down, that we need to reconnect to our roots and that we need to renew our approach to interacting with nature. This book is an important step in that direction as it flows from species to species, connecting people, nature and history. Young and old, scientists, healers, storytellers and the layperson will all take away knowledge, understanding and appreciation of the plants and natural areas around us through this book. A thoughtful, well-researched and beautifully written work such as this will be cherished by those lucky enough to view its pages.

—Scott Gillingwater

Species at Risk Biologist, Author, Educator and Naturalist

Acknowledgments

A book is never written alone, and there are so many I would like to thank. First, I would like to acknowledge my father, who encouraged me to write this book so that his grandchildren could enjoy the wisdom of these plants. Sadly, he passed into the spirit world before it was completed, but I know he would find comfort in knowing that this knowledge is not lost.

I am so appreciative for the many teachers and students who walked beside me and influenced my studies; they continue to inspire. I am deeply grateful for the loving support of my parents and grandparents, who instilled in me the magic and mysteries of nature, and I am blessed to have my mother, who gave me roots and wings and continues to nurture my spirit. As well, I need to thank my brother and sisters for the many happy journeys we shared that fostered my sense of adventure and deep love for the natural world, some of which are shared here in this book.

My deepest appreciation goes to the many wonderful children I have come to know through the years, who allow me to once again see the world through their eyes; and I will always have my heartfelt gratitude to the healing plants that bring such joy and delight to my life and are so willing to share their gifts.

Most importantly, I need to thank Rick, my partner and friend, for his steadfast support, patience and encouragement. This book would never have been completed without his help.

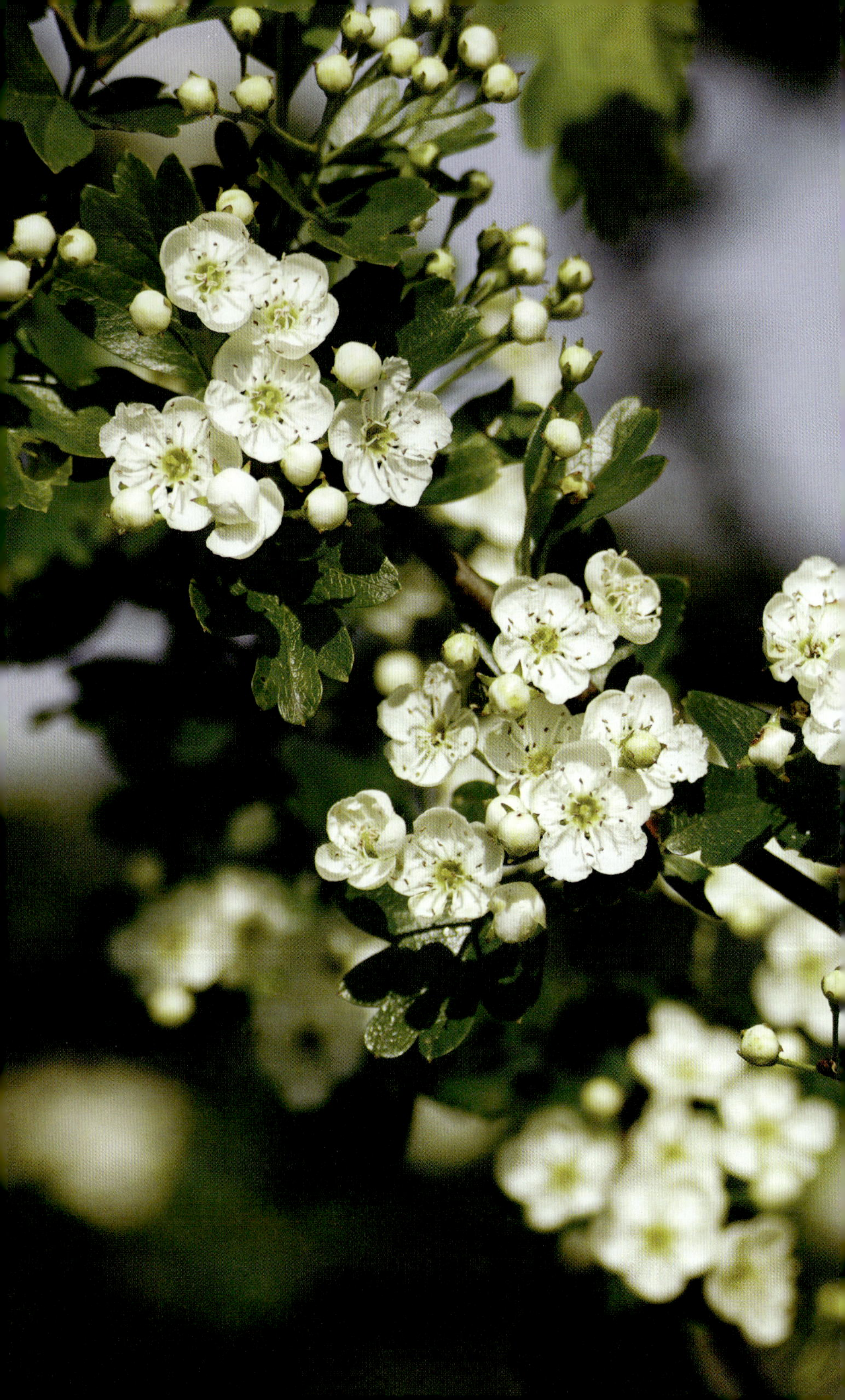

Introduction

Every tree has a story, a narrative that unfolds, slowly bringing to light its identity. Every tree has a past, a history that has been handed down from parent to child, to disclose its personality. Of all the living beings on earth, trees have remained most true to their original purpose; still following the same teachings set out for them from the beginning. It is my honour to reopen these doors and pass along their often-forgotten uses, traditions and stories.

When encountering a tree for the first time, often it is their appearance that first grabs our attention, helping us make a connection. Whether it is the flower, unique leaves, fruit or massive size, some aspect of their beauty draws us to them. Tree have played a significant role in our history, and are valued for their versatility, hardiness and beauty. They have been bestowed with gifts, and since their beginning, their aptitudes of medicine, food and utilitarian virtues have been employed to benefit people. They also have a purpose in the environment, expertly healing the earth, controlling erosion, absorbing pollutants or providing food, nesting material and cover for wildlife. They are surrounded with many myths, legends and folktales, and their amusing stories and magical uses have been passed on to generations of children.

Trees are our oldest teachers, holding a collective wisdom that awakens and strengthens the four aspects of our being — mind, body, emotions and soul. Fostering a relationship by sitting or meditating with them helps us connect with their spirit and learn from their lessons, giving us incite on different aspects of our lives.

This book is not meant to be read from cover to cover, but rather I encourage you to choose one tree, sit with it, then listen and discover its unique personality. Whether you are just starting your journey with trees or have been friends for many years, I hope these words inspire you to continue on your herbal path.

Please be aware that this information is intended to be a general guide to plant medicine and not meant to replace a professional doctor. Do not self-diagnose or self-treat for serious or long-term conditions without consulting a qualified herbalist or medical practitioner.

Basswood

Tilea americana

Linden, Linden Flower, Lime Blossom, Lime Tree, Bast Tree, Humming Tree and Bee Tree

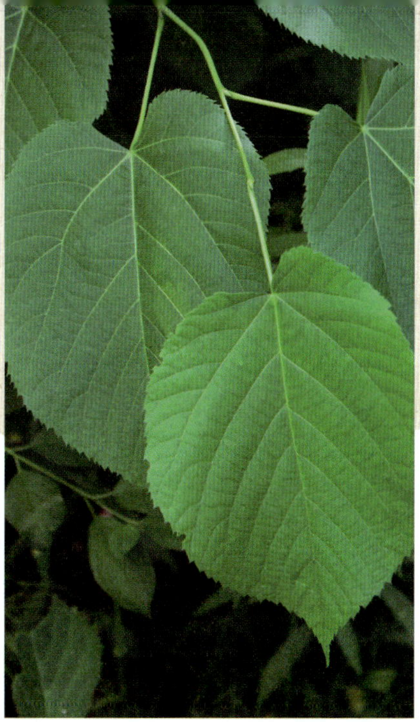

Known for its hospitality, linden's spirit is welcoming, friendly and generous. In Europe, they were customarily planted in urban centers to evoke a relaxing and calming energy, and this same tree is still regularly found along streets and in public parks, providing comfort and shade beneath its beautiful canopy.

Meeting Basswood

While little leaf linden (Tilea cordata) graces the landscape of southern England and other parts of Europe, it is its big-leaf cousin, the American basswood (Tilea americana), that inhabits the hardwood forests of eastern North America. This tree is considered a mid-tolerant species. Shade helps their seedlings get a start in life, but as they age, adequate light is required to ensure vigorous growth. Their unique, heart-shaped leaves have an asymmetrical or lopsided base and are quite large in size. Because of this characteristic, I often refer to it as the "toilet paper tree."

While in bloom, these trees are easily located by the sweet fragrance their flowers surrender. Clusters of yellowish-white florets, which produce plenty of nectar, are found dangling from narrow, ribbon-like bracts or wings. Each flower is shaped like a tiny umbrella that acts to protect the nectar from rain and morning dew. Bees adore them, and when in bloom the loud humming of bees is audible throughout forest communities, parks and neighbourhoods. Because the highly aromatic flowers draw plenty of these insects, it is sometimes known as the "humming tree" or "bee tree." The scent is believed to have an uplifting effect on the consciousness, and in folklore it was alleged that if you fell into an enchanted sleep beneath its branches, you would awake in fairyland.

Basswoods coppice readily and are frequently found growing in circular clumps where saplings have sprouted from old, remnant stumps. Because they regenerate from living roots, the aged stump is capable of living for several hundred years. An ancient stooled tree residing at Westonbirt Arboretum in Gloucestershire, England, has been estimated to be 2000 years old.

Meaning of its Name

One of basswood's most valued articles of use was its bast, a type of fiber prepared from the inner bark to make twine and cordage. The name basswood is therefore believed to be a corruption of "bast wood." The botanical name *Tilea* was derived from the Greek word *ptilon,* meaning winged, denoting the large leaf-like bract from which the flower stalks, and later the fruit, arise. In Europe it is often known as lime or lime blossom; however, this name has caused confusion, since it is not related in any way to the lime tree in the citrus family.

In the Garden

The energy of basswood is soft and comforting to the heart, making this beautiful tree a wonderful addition to gardens. The large leaves, which form a cool, protective canopy, offer us shade from the summer heat. They can be incorporated into fragrant gardens, and because both the leaves and flowers are non-toxic to children, they are a good choice for playground plantings. Being very high in sugary nectar, the sweet blossoms are valued by beekeepers.

Wildlife Value

Basswood provides many gifts to the forest community. The fragrant flower produces copious amounts of pollen and nectar. Because they hang like umbrellas, they allow easy access to bumblebees and other flying insects, making them an important food source for our native pollinators. The downy, pea-size fruit, which are produced in large numbers in autumn, afford nourishment to upland game birds, songbirds, foxes, squirrels, chipmunks and other small rodents, and the twigs and leaves are enjoyed by a variety of mammals, including cottontails, deer and porcupines. Small, continuous holes resembling necklaces around the circumfer-

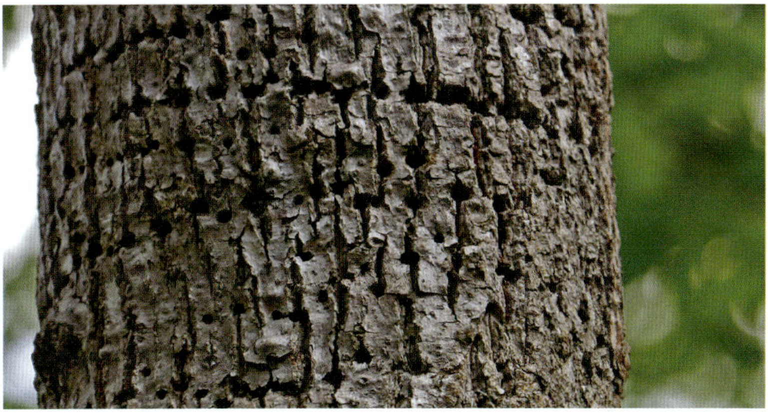

Sapsucker holes in bark

ence of the trunk are a sign that yellow-bellied sapsuckers were in the area feeding.

Basswoods also offer shelter for various woodland species. The soft wood is favoured by woodpeckers for making their nesting cavities, and these in turn are reused in subsequent years by secondary cavity-users unable to excavate their own holes. These successive users, including saw-whet owls, wood ducks, great crested flycatchers and nuthatches, rely on either naturally occurring cavities, where a rotting limb has broken, or holes excavated by other birds. As years pass, the dens continue to provide a succession of homes and are exploited by porcupines, raccoons, flying squirrels and swarms of honeybees. Ring-necked snakes will lay their eggs in the base of old, hollow basswoods, especially when subjected to warm sunlight.

Culinary Uses

Herbal tea made from the flowers is one of the most widely used beverages in Europe, where it is drunk daily for its pleasant taste and health benefits. It is commonly available in grocery stores in Canada and often sold as linden or lime blossom tea. Sipping the warm brew in the evening is relaxing, and a cold infusion makes a delightful cooling drink on hot, summer days. The edible flowers were traditionally served with fruit and desserts, and when picked in early spring, the young leaves are eaten as a salad green. In winter, the bright red buds, which are slightly mucilaginous and taste similar to nuts, can be consumed as a trailside nibble.

It is maintained that the white honey made from the nectar of linden flowers is of the finest quality, having an exquisite minty flavor.

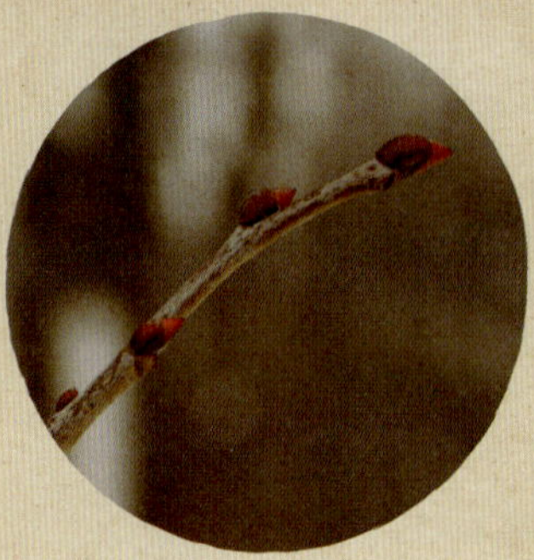

Basswood twig in winter

It is particularly used in making liqueurs and prevalent in the wine industry.

Medicinal Uses

It is the flowers that provide the medicinal properties, found in both our native basswood and the little leaf linden, and can be enjoyed in tea, cordial or infused honey. The actions are moistening and cooling and, because of its pleasant taste and gentle effects, it makes a wonderful remedy for children and the elderly. Its mild, relaxing properties provide an outstanding sedative used to strengthen the heart, calm the nervous system and induce sleep.

The flowers and bracts are collected when the blossoms are just opening. Their potency quickly dissipates when dried and stored, so it is best to use them within a few months of harvesting.

Calming Nervine

French herbalist Maurice Messegue (1921-2017) called linden the "tea of happiness." This remedy was best known for its relaxing qualities and continues to be purchased as a calming tea. Due to its mild, sedative action on the nerves, it makes a perfect remedy for reducing stress and nervous tension. It gently soothes anxiety and panic attacks by calming the heart and quieting the mind. During the Second World War, it was a recommended beverage in Britain when cities were under attack.

Linden is also one of the most effective herbs for insomnia, particularly when caused by stress, nervousness or irritation of the mind. By relieving tension, it encourages a restful and relaxing sleep, leaving one refreshed in the morning. This gentle remedy is also ideal for calming overactive or restless children before bed, helping them settle at night.

Cardiovascular Health

The heart-shaped leaves seem to point to linden's affinity to the heart. It has been reputed as a calming heart tonic, and its mild astringent, antispasmodic and vasodilator properties have been shown to have a cooling, toning and relaxing effect on the cardiovascular system. By dilating the blood vessels and relaxing the arteries, it helps to let go of constraint and tension. This improves circulation and brings more nourishment and support to the heart, thereby making the entire system more efficient.

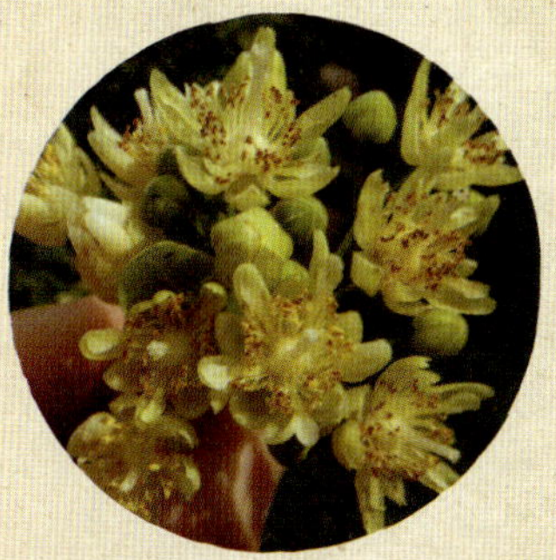

Basswood flowers provide medicinal benefits

Rich in antioxidants, linden effectively quells raised blood pressure and heart palpitations, specifically when stress, anxiety and nervous tension are contributing factors. As well, new research shows that it may be helpful for protecting the heart and reducing arteriosclerosis by lowering blood cholesterol levels, thinning the blood and removing fatty deposits in the blood vessels.

Cold and Flu Remedy

Linden is valued for feverish colds and flus, particularly benefiting children. Sweating is the system's natural way of preventing a fever from burning too hot, while at the same time helping eliminate toxins through the pores in the skin or clearing them through the kidneys. A hot linden tea has a slight diaphoretic action that promotes perspiration, thereby assisting to reduce the temperature of the body and "breaking a fever."

Its mucilage content also helps soothe inflamed and irritated respiratory passages, sore throats, and dry coughs. Furthermore, it boosts the immune system, thus helping the body to become more resistant to infections.

Cosmetic Uses

The warm, honey-like aroma of linden flowers make them a popular fragrance in perfumes and soaps and the essential oil is often sold under the name "tilleul." The flowers and leaves are used in baths to help regenerate and refresh tired, dull skin and are included in facial rinses to clear freckles and wrinkles.

Bois Blanc

The early French Canadians referred to basswood as *bois blanc*, which means white wood. Being very soft and lightweight, it is valued by carvers because it is easy to work and sands readily. The fine, straight grain and white colouring allows it to take on supreme sharpness and minute details. This made it specific for carving intricate pieces of art. The light wood also made functional shields during the Middle Ages.

Basswood continues to be an important commercial wood that is used for small articles not requiring strength or durability. It is commonly turned into bowls or made into wooden kitchen wares, splints, toys and other novelties. Because it has no odour or taste, it was traditionally utilized in items for making and storing food, such as bread bins, food containers and butter churns. Its light weight and good acoustic properties make it suitable for crafting musical instruments such as guitar bodies, woodwinds and drum shells. It produces good-quality pulp and excelsior for packaging, and its veneer is used for baskets. It holds little value for outdoor use since it rots quickly once wet, and when employed as fuel, it produces little heat.

Fibre Source

The Indigenous people used the bast to produce essential fiber. When the inner bark was soaked in water for two to four weeks, the long, fibrous strands could easily be loosened and separated from the softer, woody tissue. They were then twisted and plied into suitable twine, cordage and rope for fishing nets, snowshoe netting, coarse matting and storage bags for food. They used it to tie their poles together to make the framework of their shelters and longhouses, and many tribes valued it for sewing shoes, clothing, birch bark dishes and berry baskets.

Because basswood twine was easy to handle and soft on the hands, it was soon favoured by the early pioneers, and it became customary to have a ball of basswood string in every household. The strong fibers also made suitable brushes for spreading paint, glue and pitch.

Tree of Love and Immortality

Linden is a feminine tree, sacred to Venus and associated with Freyja, the motherly goddess of truth and love. This tree aligns with matters of the heart, and the heart-shaped leaves are considered a sign pointing to these attributes. In German folklore, linden is the tree of lovers. Courtships were started beneath its boughs, and talismans of love were made from the wood. It is specifically known as the tree of conjugal love (united in marriage) and fidelity, and wedding vows were said under its canopy to bring marital happiness.

It was considered the tree of immortality, and to grow a basswood on your property ensured your family tree would continue. This tree brings blessings to new babies, and ceremonial plantings were common to mark the birth of a child or other special family events.

Tree of Tranquility, Truth and Grace

Basswood's bright spirit was believed to bring tranquility to domestic or family issues. They were planted in front of churches and in the heart of villages, where they could be present in everyday life. Traditionally, local communities would assemble under the trees to dance, celebrate, commune and hold social gatherings. Here too, local leaders would conduct their meetings to make decisions on matters of common interest or public business. The tree came to represent the tongue of honesty and clear sight. Because it was be-

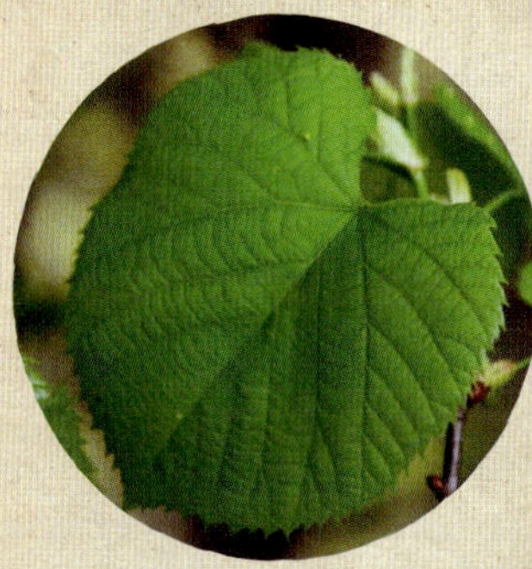

The heart-shaped leaf points to the heart

lieved to unearth the truth and restore justice and peace, it was also associated with judgment, and in rural Germany, court verdicts were announced sub-tilea, or *under the linden.*

Since basswood became a symbol of truth and grace, it was believed that it was impossible to tell a lie while standing beneath it. When people assembled under its peaceful canopy, it encouraged them to communicate with respect, kindness and humility and allowed one to retain composure in any situation.

The Tree of Sweetness and Blessings

The calming energy of basswood brings comfort to the heart and drives away ill-meaning spirits that can carry impairment. It was believed that dragons came to rest in its shade so no harm could manifest. These could have been mythological dragons but were more likely a metaphor for grieving, depression and sadness. As a calming nervine, basswood assists in alleviating nervous and emotional worries.

Lessons of Basswood

This tree brings blessings and sweetness into your life, and sitting under a basswood helps you to realize them. When faced with tough decisions or when life is pulling you in different directions, it can help redirect and guide you down the right path. This transpires by searching deep within your heart and allowing basswood to bring to light life's potential.

Beech

Fagus grandifolia

Beechnut Tree and Love Tree

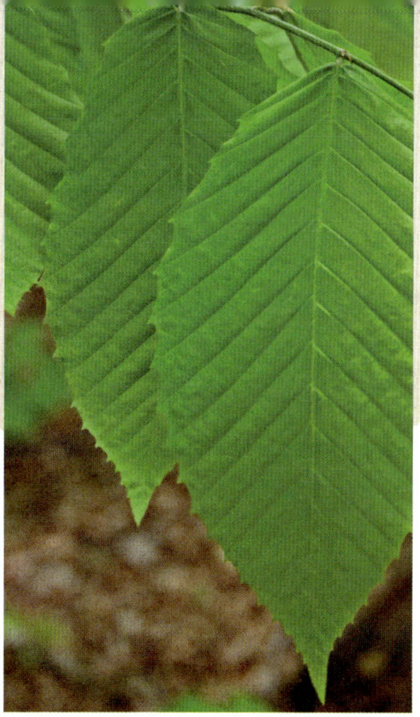

The most striking attribute of beech is her regal presence. Tall and elegant, with feminine contours, she casts ample shade onto the forest floor due to her vast crown and grand size. When growing in open areas, her branches extend close to the ground, but in a woodland setting, they are held high, emphasizing her tall, graceful trunk. The vertical boles, which rise like columns, not only depict strength and stability, but also portray tranquility and solitude. The lofty interior of beech forests has often been compared to the inside of a church, and it is rumoured that early gothic cathedrals were inspired by beech groves. The sacred energy of beech continues to be revered, and it is believed that prayers uttered beneath her boughs go directly to heaven.

Like white birch, beech has a strong female presence in the forest, and while birch is the "lady," she is the "queen." She stands as a stately feminine consort to the oak king, and at Summer Solstice her wood is burnt with oak, symbolizing their relationship. She is also often considered the "mother of the woods," and her generous, protective and nurturing spirit offers shade, food and seclusion to those in her embrace.

Meeting Beech

One of beech's most distinctive features is the smooth, bluish-gray bark. It has a certain resemblance to an elephant's leg and can't help invite touch to those passing. Beech groves were once thought to be full of mystery and menace. Spots and fissures in the bark, where branches have fallen off, form eye-shaped scars and at dusk may conjure up ideas that the forest is watching you. Some people felt beech forests were unlucky plac-

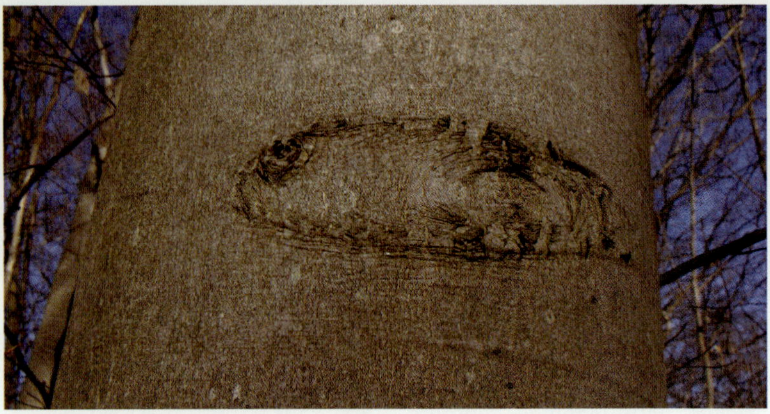

Eye-shaped scars on bark

es to be found alone at night and that the scars represented the "evil eye"; others considered beeches to be enchanted trees and the protective eyes played the role of watching for danger. Nonetheless, in Europe, these forests inspired a rich tradition and were the setting for many folktales, including Grimm's fairy tales, Tolkien's Hobbit, and stories of Robin Hood and his merry men.

As the botanical name *grandifolia* indicates, American beech foliage is larger than others in the beech genus. When unfolding, the copper-coloured leaves have silky hairs, but become green and take on a leathery texture as they mature. By fall they turn a deep, golden-rust. Sheltered young trees in the understory hold onto their papery leaves throughout winter, which bleach to ivory white as the season progresses. In spring, the canopy is light and airy, allowing a show of ephemeral woodland flowers; however, during the summer months the massive crown, which becomes quite dense, permits little light to the forest floor, and undergrowth is sparse.

Male and female flowers develop on the same tree and appear soon after the leaves emerge. Wind assists pollination, and the female flower matures into a pair of triangular nuts enclosed in a bristly, reddish-brown case. When ripe, the casing splits into four parts to reveal the fruit, which is commonly dispersed by birds and mammals. A good seed crop usually occurs every three to five years.

Growing Habits

Beech trees are slow growing and can live three to four hundred years. In Europe, the European beech was commonly coppiced. This traditional management practice involved repeatedly cutting a tree near ground level to encourage new shoots to emerge from the stump. In subsequent years, the young growth was harvested for poles or firewood and the cycle would begin again. Coppicing maintains the trees at a juvenile stage so that they rarely die of old age; therefore, some coppice stumps can reach exceptional maturity, and many have been estimated at over 1000 years.

American beech grows best on rich, loamy soils with good drainage. Its presence often indicates a diversity of flora and fauna, and early settlers looked for large, healthy trees as a sign of fertile farmland. Like many trees, beech relies heavily on symbiotic relationships with various soil fungi, known as mycorrhiza, to pass minerals to the roots in exchange for sugars and nutrients from the tree. Mycorrhiza also act as an underground communication network, allowing the trees to exchange chemical "information" and share resources below ground, even with different species. Through these organisms, trees in a forest are able to support each other and assist those that are sick or in distress.

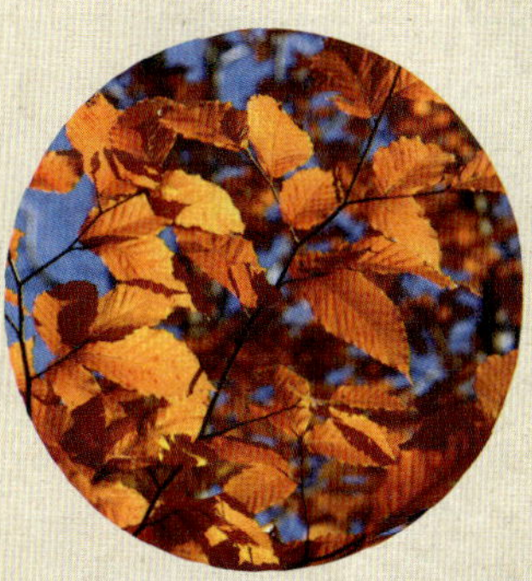

Golden colour of leaves in fall

Beech seedlings are very shade tolerant, and this tree is one of the few species that grows well in low light. They seem quite happy to wait in the shadow of their mother as she nurtures and helps them along. For years, they survive in the understory, and after another succumbs to disease or old age, they make their way into the canopy. Biding its time when young actually benefits the tree in the future. This slower growth produces tighter wood, making the tree more resistant to fungi as it ages, thus affording a longer life.

In Europe, beech trees can be seen lining laneways of affluent estates, which seems fitting, since beech boughs are a symbol of prosperity.

Mysterious Shapes

Although very shade tolerant, beech is also highly light responsive, and even a small difference in sun filtering through the canopy influences growth. The slightest change in light intensity can pull the tree in one direction or another, which often accounts for many crooked trunks and twisted branches. The elegant contours were though to resemble spirits emerging from the earth, which inspired many mysterious tales. In Medieval Europe, trees were held in high regard. It was believed that tree spirits resided in them, thus they were never damaged or destroyed. Beech trees were not the only trees honoured for housing dryads. Groves of oak and ash also provided protection and were considered to be some of the oldest sanctuaries.

Circles of Beech

Beech roots are comprised of a deep tap root, which keeps the tree upright in wind storms, and shallow horizontal roots that are easily observed growing just above the soil surface. These unprotected roots are susceptible to drought and mechanical damage from vehicles or equipment. While seedlings readily germinate from beechnuts, most beech stands colonize by vegetative means. New saplings arise from the exposed surface roots of their mother, and when she dies, a circle of young trees remains. At one time, it was believed that strong magical energies could be felt within these rings.

Beech Drops

Associated with American beech is an odd little plant known as beech drops (*Epifagus virginiana*). They can be found growing beneath the tree yet are often overlooked because, instead of being green, they are brown, similar to the fallen leaves on the forest floor. This plant does not possess chlorophyll, but instead is parasitic to beech roots and depends on the tree for energy and nourishment. The scientific name *Epifagus* means "upon the beech."

Bark Carvings

The bark is tempting to anyone toting a pocket knife, enticing them to carve their initials on the smooth surface. Today, many disapprove of the graffiti; however, writing messages on beech bark is an ancient custom dating back to ancient Rome and was considered a way of honouring those who passed before. Lovers favoured carving their affections into the trunks so that their love would grow with the tree. Because of this tradition, the beech is sometimes known as the "love tree," and in the *Language of Flowers* it came to symbolize a lover's tryst. This practice can be verified by the survival of an ancient Latin expression "crescent illae, crescetis amores" meaning as these letters grow, so may our love. Carving on trees was also noted in Shakespeare's play *As You Like It*, when Orlando says, "O Rosalind! These trees shall be my books, find in their barks my thoughts I'll character." Such documentation is made possible due to the rapid formation of cork cambium that quickly seals the wounds, allowing the scars to remain visible for years.

The First Writing Surface

The connection between this tree and writing is ancient and the smooth boles of beech trees provided one of the earliest writing surfaces. It has been suggested the words *book* and *beech* were derived from common linguistic roots. The Anglo-Saxon word for beech is *boc*, which later became *book*. This association is evident in many languages, including German and Swedish. Due to the close grain in the wood, which gives a smooth even surface, beech runic tablets were commonly written on and thin slices of the wood were bound together to form the first books. Words inscribed on beech were considered to take on power; therefore, beech tablets were held in high regards.

Wildlife Value

Beechnuts, also known as beech mast, provide a significant food source for a great number of critters. Not only do deer feed on them greedily, various birds, such as wood ducks, wild turkeys, grouses, and pigeons, also take great delight in eating them. The nuts are a vital food for squirrels and chipmunks, which are so dependent on them that if there is a meagre harvest a visible decline in their population may be noticed. Mice have been known to layup four to eight quarts of carefully shelled nuts in a safe log or hollow tree.

Black bears are also heavy beechnut consumers. Bears don't wait for a meal to drop to the forest floor, but instead go right to the source at the top of the tree. Here, they often leave messy accumulations of dead, broken branches called bear "nests." In the fall, they climb high into tree crotches, and as they reach out to pull nut-laden branches towards them, many of the branches are partially broken. The result is a tangle of sticks that, from the ground, resemble a huge nest.

Beech leaves have a tendency to remain dry and springy even in moist weather and are favoured by squirrels for building a leaf nest in a crotch or for lining their winter homes.

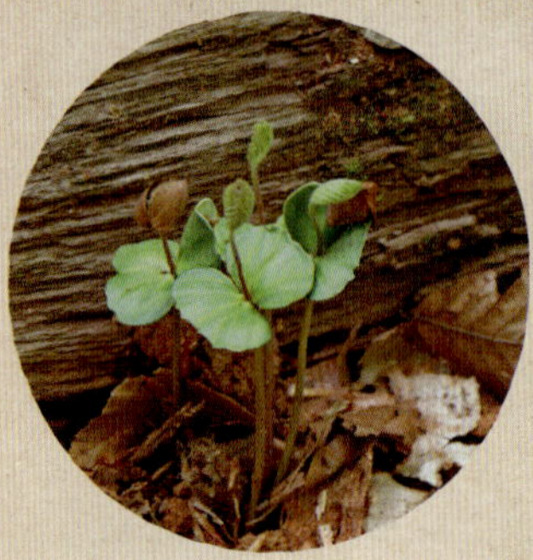

Beech seedling from seed germination

Passenger Pigeons

The now-extinct passenger pigeon was once an integral part of the ecology of beech, and these trees in turn provided them a staple food. The birds doted on nuts, including beechnuts, hickory nuts, acorns and chestnuts, consuming high numbers when available. Once described as being in countless numbers, their populations, according to modern ornithologists, reached three to five billion during the sixteenth century. Thousands would descend on beech trees, devouring their sweet nuts. They roosted in such great numbers that branches would break, and later, the birds were equally destructive to telegraph wires. So abundant, they formed a major part of colonial diets, and overhunting and habitat loss from clearing the forests are believed to be the two major factors in their demise. A series of crop failures may also have contributed to decreasing populations, causing them to go extinct by the early 1900s. The final passenger pigeon (Martha) died in the summer of 1914.

The Elders of our Society

In trees, the living portion exists just under the bark and the center is made up of dead material. Therefore, even when a trunk is void of inner wood, these trees can still develop healthy crowns and continue to live for decades. While hollow trees are not as structurally sound as their younger counterparts and offer little lumber value to loggers, they still provide an essential role in the forest ecosystem, making excellent wildlife dens and nesting cavities.

Beech trees can live for many centuries, and these elders are important members of the forest society. Each year these magnificent giants afford homes, shelter and roosting sites for birds, bats, squirrels, raccoons and other forms of wildlife. Watching a new batch of young get their start in a beech tree is an enjoyable experience.

Culinary Uses

The scientific name *Fagus* comes from the Greek word *phagus*, meaning to eat, and most likely referenced the edible nut. Like walnuts, acorns and hazelnuts, beechnuts were once a valuable inclusion in the diets of the First Nations people, to augment their agricultural crops and hunting. The early settlers also gathered the fallen nuts after the first frosty night in October to store for winter use. So popular, that in the early 1900s the nuts could be found in Boston and New York markets when in season. Early pioneers also turned to the beech forest to fatten their hogs and turkeys on the fallen mast, and pigs that were fed beechnuts and acorns were believed to produce the best-tasting pork.

The triangular nuts are encased in a prickly shell and when split open release their tasty contents. The sweet and nutritious kernels are small and difficult to extract from their leathery covering, but once freed, they are delicious roasted and can be eaten as is, used as a coffee substitute or ground into beechnut butter. As well as containing 22% protein, they also have a high percentage of fat, affording outstanding oil from the pressed kernel. This was used for cooking and as lamp oil.

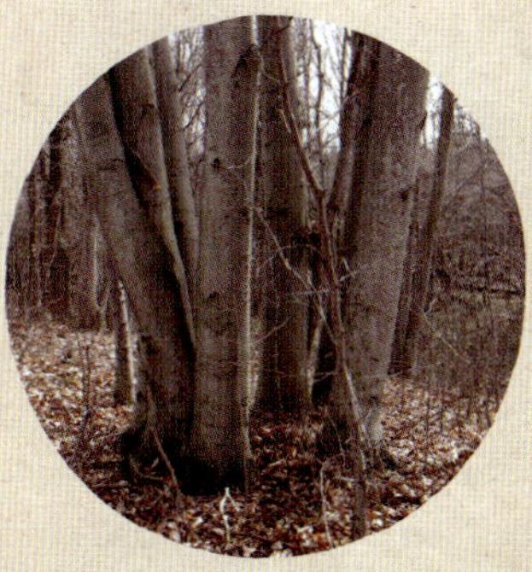

Circle of beech trees

The tender, spring leaves are edible and when mixed with other greens make a nice addition to salads. The young leaves were also steeped in gin for several weeks and then sweetened to produce a light, greenish-yellow liqueur known a beech-leaf noyau.

Beech wood is used to smoke herring, Westphalian ham, various sausages and certain cheeses. Beech logs are also burned to dry the malt used in some German smoked beers, giving them their unique flavour. Chips of beech wood continue to be used in brewing Budweiser beer as a fining agent. This compound is added to beer near the completion of the fermenting process to help improve clarity and to adjust the flavour and aroma.

Essence of Beech

Bach flower remedies, developed by Edward Bach in the 1930s, use diluted dew from the flowers to leave an energetic signature of the plant. According to the system, beech is for those who are intolerant, arrogant, lack humility, find fault and blame in others, are critical and lack sympathy. It is used to promote acceptance, patience and an easygoing attitude, and helps to boost confidence and hope.

Wood Value

As lumber, beech is unsuitable for major construction projects or fence posts, as it has a tendency to warp during seasoning and rots quickly when coming in contact with soil. However, the strong, hard wood has a fine grain and is knot-free, making it appropriate for small articles such as tool handles, carpenter planes, stonemason's mallets, granary shovels and wooden cogs for water wheels.

Another unique feature of beech wood is that it is odourless and tasteless. This characteristic, plus the fact the hard wood resists knife cuts, brought about its common application as chopping blocks and cutting boards. It was also used for food containers, butter churns, butter tubs, buckets to hold maple sap, food bowls, and wooden spoons.

For domestic fuel, there is hardly any better firewood. It is easily split, smokeless, clean burning, provides strong heat for many hours, and offers a bright but calm flame.

Other Uses

Beech leaves were once used to fill mattresses because they were devoid of a musky smell and gave a certain springy comfort that was lacking in straw. In France these beds were known as *lilts de parlement*, or speaking beds. Furthermore, even on damp days, the unshed winter leaves stay dry; thus, they can be gathered and stuffed into coats to warm a person who gets caught in the cold or used to start fires and line winter shelters.

Artists from the seventeenth and eighteenth century collected soot from chimneys after burning beech wood and mixed it with water to make a dark grey pigment with a hint of yellow. This ink was known as "soot brown" or *bistre.* The papery leaves clinging to winter branches are beautiful in handmade paper and children gather beechnuts to thread into necklaces.

Protection from Lightning

The beech tree is believed to possess natural protection from lightning strikes and was planted near homes to safeguard dwellings from adverse weather. This superstition actually has some truth to it, since, when compared with other trees, the beech is statistically struck by lightning less often, or at least receives little harm when it draws the heavenly flurry. The reason for this is that the high oil content in the wood and the thin, flat bark is reputed to resist electricity. As moisture runs down the smooth trunk, it creates a continuous sheet of water. When lightning strikes, the electricity travels down the outside of the trees into the earth and damage is minimal. If you are curious as to which tree is struck by lightning most often; the consensus is the oak. Oak's thick, rough bark causes the rain water to cascade and form hundreds of tiny water falls; thus, the flow of electricity is continuously interrupted, causing injury to the tree if a lightning bolt should strike.

The Tree of Wisdom and Knowledge

For the Druids, beech was considered the tree of knowledge and wisdom and was strongly associated with books, learning and human intellect. Because of this connection, it is said to contain ancient knowledge and innate wisdom that has accumulated for many generations, and is considered to hold the totality of insight and perception of all other trees. It symbolizes the written word and the transmission of lore, and reminds us of the importance of early teachings and the significance of preserving our knowledge to benefit future generations. We have an obligation to realize this wisdom and pass it down to our children.

As the holder of this vast amount of knowledge and wisdom, the beech was able to truly reach out to humans and share her lessons. She grants access to those who ask for it and who honour and acknowledge her presence. The manifestation of her spirit is thought to be personified in the rustling of her leaves.

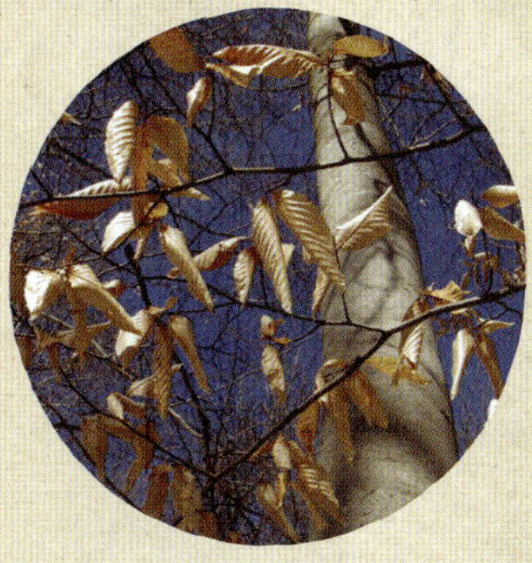

The dried leaves remain on the branches through winter

Folklore

The smooth bark is a nice canvas upon which to design; thus, a talisman of beech wood was carried to increase creative energy. Furthermore, it had the ability to bring luck and success to the bearer, and a small piece in your right shoe might lead you to fortune. Water collected at dawn from pools in the hollows of ancient beeches was believed to have great healing benefits. Falling asleep and dreaming under beech boughs would ensure your dreams would come true.

In Celtic mythology, beech was known as the "tree of wishes," and a fallen branch was considered an invitation from the wishing fairies. Scratching or carving a wish onto a beech stick was said to make it come true, if it was to be. Once written upon, the stick was buried in the ground and the wish would be manifested as the wood decayed and was reabsorbed back into the earth.

Lessons of Beech

As the tree of wisdom and understanding, beech has many lessons to provide. She increases our capacity for learning and inspires a thirst for knowledge. By turning to beech, we connect with our ancestral past, so we can rediscover lost wisdom. This deep knowledge, passed down through time, helps provide a firm foundation on which to build new ideas and make healthy decisions in our lives. Guidance from the past can gain insight into the future and help us move forward.

In spring, beech requires a great deal of energy to simultaneously form new leaves and shed the old. This power is bestowed on us to give us inner strength and confidence, thereby allowing us to see ourselves in a more positive light, freeing us from our inner fears and enabling us to express ourselves more confidently. It assists us in resolving conflict by radiating calmness and self-assurance and provides us the tools to make good decisions and form honorable opinions.

Just as the branches are drawn towards the sun, beech teaches us that sometimes we need to follow the light within our heart. The eyes fixed in the trunk continuously watch over us with love and protection and remind us to see the good in all people and recognize there is a positive lesson in every situation. Like the new generation of beech trees circling around their mother, we are all part of a community, living, loving and working together. If we get disconnected, it is like an ember becoming separated from the fire; the light within quickly burns out.

Black Cherry

Prunus serotina

Wild Black Cherry, Rum Cherry, Bird Cherry

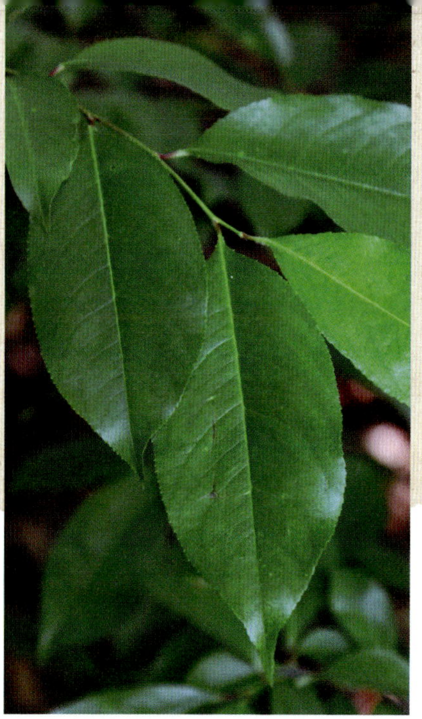

Growing up, we had a large tree at the back of our property where my father suspended a swing from one of its branches. My grandmother revealed to me that my special tree was a black cherry. She showed me how to identify it by its distinctive flaky bark that resembles burnt cornflakes. My grandfather, in his humorous way, remarked that "you put black cherries on your burnt cornflakes in the morning," and I still use this analogy when hiking with children to help them recognize this beautiful tree.

Meeting Black Cherry

Black cherry, a tree native to the deciduous forest of eastern North America, is a member of the rose family and known as the "blooming lady." It is prized in our landscape for its fragrant blossoms in early spring and colourful fruit later in the season. The young trees are somewhat shade tolerant; however, in full sun, they thrive and grow quickly, colonizing openings and edges of woodlands. This makes them an ideal choice for naturalization projects. As they age, more sun is required for them to successfully rise into the canopy. To keep their place in the forest ecosystem they often depend on the demise of another tree to ensure adequate light.

Black cherry is considered the largest cherry species in the world, growing 25 meters (80 feet) or more in height and obtaining a diameter of 1.2 meters (4 feet). They usually survive 80 to 100 years; however, it is not uncommon to find them reaching an age of 150 to 200 years. The mature tree is easily recognized in any season, even from a distance, as the dark, flaky bark stands out among the trunks of other trees. The foliage turns an outstanding bright yellow with slight orange hues in fall as temperatures begin to decrease.

The small, white flowers appear in long, drooping masses or racemes in early spring when the leaves are new. Known as progressive bloomers, the blossoms begin emerging at the bottom of the cluster and work upwards. This trait ensures that if a drop in temperature destroys early blooms, subsequent flowers will allow the tree to set fruit. When fully open, they are pollinated by insects; however, self-fertilization can occur when specialized pollinators, such as bees and beetles, are not available. In summer, each string of flowers is succeeded by a grape-like bunch of small, juicy fruit. The ripe cherries are purple-black, about the size of peas, and have a sour taste. The soft flesh surrounds a hard seed or pit, which can remain viable in the soil for many years. When eaten by birds and mammals, they are dispersed in their droppings, thus aiding in the tree's distribution. Studies have shown that passing through digestive tracts improves the seed's rate of germination.

Wildlife Value

The flowers, leaves and fruit of black cherry attract and feed many forms of wildlife, and when established in the landscape, this tree helps increase beneficial insect and songbird populations. Generous in both nectar and pollen, cherries are valued by native bees, bumblebees and honeybees, and their buzzing is audible in spring as they visit the flowers.

Although the leaves contain toxic compounds, black cherry feeds a staggering number of insects and is a primary food source for many butterfly and moth (*Lepidoptera*) larvae. Red spotted purple butterfly, viceroy, eastern tiger swallowtail butterfly, Cecropia moth, polyphemus moth and sphinx moth are among the various species that lay their eggs on the shiny leaves. The cyanide-generating chemicals found in the tree may provide important value to these *Lepidoptera* species. The toxins, when taken up by the growing caterpillars, are possibly used as a means of protection from predators or employed later in their life as colour pigment in their wings. The caterpillars also attract many birds, such as the yellow and black billed cuckoo and northern oriole, which feed on them.

With the ripening of fruit come numerous birds. Cherries generously share their berries with seventy

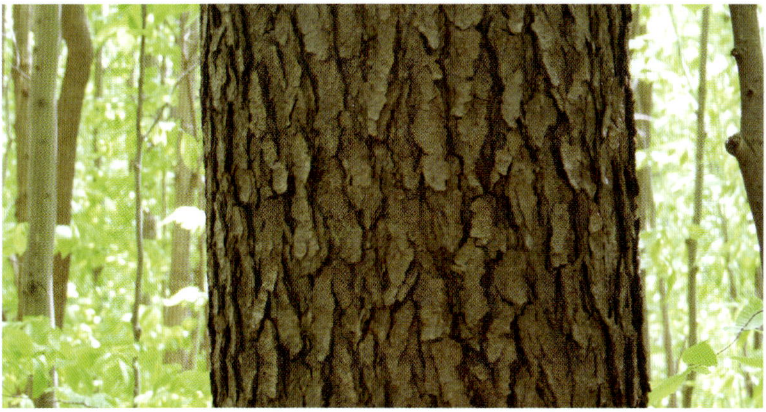

Black cherry's distinctive bark resembles cornflakes

or more bird species. Occasionally, birds become intoxicated on the overripe fruit that ferments late in the season. Birds that have overconsumed such cherries will have uncertain balance and glazed eyes.

Mammals, including mice, chipmunks, squirrels, cottontails, opossums, raccoons and foxes, also frequently feast on the fruit. Indeed, bears are so fond of black cherries that they can be quite determined to succeed in obtaining them. These "cherry bears," as they were referred to by the early pioneers, were particularly feisty individuals and best left alone.

Birds such as chickadees, woodpeckers and nuthatches cache seeds and look for insects in the rough bark. The nuthatch hangs upside down while descending the trunk, efficiently searching for insects concealed in the bark crevices, while the brown creeper works in the opposite direction, circling up the trunk probing for hidden treasure.

A Favourite in Murder Mysteries

Black cherry twigs, bark, pits and foliage, particularly when damaged or wilted due to frost, drought or trampling, contain cyanogenic glycoside, which when broken down converts to a toxic compound known as hydrogen cyanide or prussic acid. All members in the *Prunus* group generate this chemical, and the scraped twig or crushed leaf will release the distinctive "bitter almond" odour telling of the toxins. Cyanide is a powerful poison that, when added to tea cups, has played a part in many murder mysteries. Within minutes after a person has ingested a lethal dose, it paralyzes the respiratory system by interfering with the cells' ability to

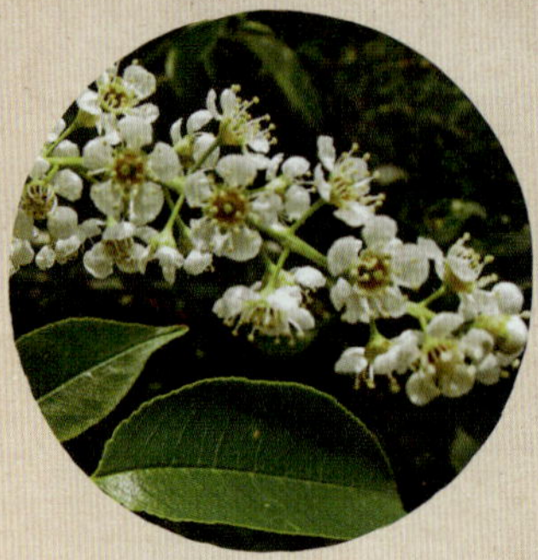

Black cherries are progressive bloomers

use oxygen, and the tissues quickly begin to "suffocate." Fortunately, only a small amount of these poisons is found in cherry, and indeed many of its therapeutic actions can be attributed to its cyanogens.

Culinary Uses

William Wood wrote that the native cherry was "so furre the mouth that the tongue will cleave to the roof." Here, he was most likely referring to our native choke cherry (*Prunus virginiana*), which, as the name implies, has an acrid taste. There is no doubt that our best native cherry for eating is the wild black or rum cherry (*Prunus serotina*), and you have to be quick to beat the birds to the crop. The fruit contains potent antioxidants and is a good source of vitamins. Although they are somewhat disappointing, being small in comparison to domestic cherries, they do have a long history of being eaten raw, cooked or dried. They are quite tart, but the addition of sugar to improve their flavour transforms them into excellent wild cherry jelly, and the early colonists cooked them into sauces, syrups and chutneys. Indigenous people also consumed the berries fresh, or dried them to add to winter soups and stews. They were essential in pemmican (pulverized lean, dry meat, mixed with berries and melted fat), which provided them vitamins, protein and fat through the winter months.

Wild cherries were used extensively to make wines, liqueurs and cordials. They were also infused in whiskey, rum and brandy to give the alcohol an agreeable flavour, and this brought to light the common name "rum cherry." Homemade cherry brandy, also known as cherry bounce, made with domestic sour cherries was reportedly one of Queen Victoria's favourite beverages. After immigrating to North America, the colonialists made their own version with native black cherries. Recipes usually instructed that the cherries be mashed, cracking the stones and all, before fermentation. This imparted a small amount of cyanide, adding a tasty touch of poison to the final product. This beverage often made a man tipsy, and to be "cherry merry" was to be riotously drunk.

Medicinal Uses

The North American Indigenous people used black cherry bark as medicine, and by the late nineteenth century it became one of the most commonly used domestic remedies in pioneer homes. Cherry's medicinal virtues benefit the digestive tract and circulation system; however, its main therapeutic actions lie in its expectorant, anti-tussive and antispasmodic properties and is primarily used for irritating coughs and as a coolant to reduce fevers. Its effectiveness as a sedative and cough suppressant is attributed to the toxic cyanogen content in the inner bark known as prussic acid, and cherry's distinctive fragrance and bitter flavour is telling of this chemical.

The cyanogenic glycoside is most abundant in fall and winter, when the medicine is traditionally collected. With a sharp knife, peel away strips of bark from young branches so minimal damage is incurred to the tree, then separate the thin, greenish inner bark from the reddish outer bark. Once it is dehydrated, store it in airtight containers protected from light. The therapeutic properties deteriorate greatly if kept longer than a year, making it necessary to collect fresh each season.

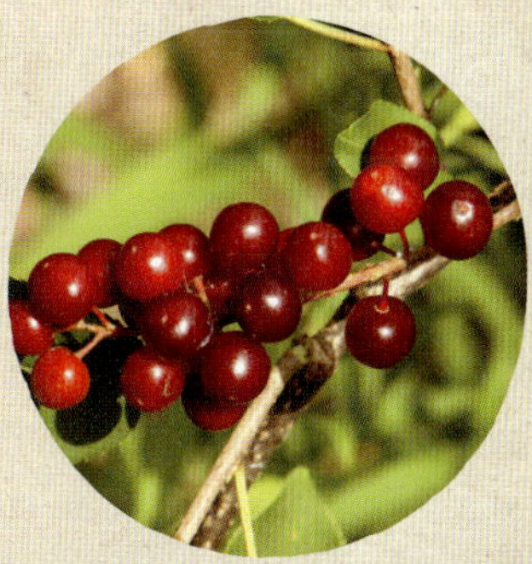

Choke cherry fruit has an acrid taste

To release the medicine, soak the inner bark in cool water for 12 to 24 hours until the "bitter almond" smell is noticeable. Boiling or overheating destroys the cyanide and impairs the medicinal properties. The longer the herb is left, the more bitter and astringent it becomes. Add alcohol to the infusion to make a tincture or formulate into syrup as a pleasant cough suppressant. It blends nicely, both in taste and action, with honey. Because the bark contains cyanide, this remedy should not be used in large or frequent doses.

Coughs

Historically, black cherry was primarily used for treating coughs. To this day, authentic wild cherry cough syrup and lozenges are made from an extract of the inner bark, and this time-honoured herb is still found in various commercial cough remedies. In small quantities, the cyanogenic glycosides have a mild sedative action on the respiratory nerves to help suppress or calm coughs. The compound quickly enters the lungs, helping to relax spasms in the smooth muscles that line the bronchioles, thereby quieting the cough reflex.

As a beneficial expectorant, cherry is recommended for treating mucus congestion, whooping cough, pneumonia, bronchitis and old, lingering coughs after an infection has passed. However, due to its antispasmodic actions, it has a particular ability to ease lung spasms or treat dry, irritable or persistent coughs caused by nervousness or an injury. Although a cough is a normal and helpful process to help remove mucus from the lungs, black cherry is an effective remedy when coughing is spasmodic and relentless, making sleep difficult. It is specifically called for when a cough is clearly counterproductive and an antitussive (anti-cough) remedy is justified.

Cooling Inflammation and Fevers

Classified as a coolant, black cherry is a principal remedy for reducing heat and irritation that results in redness, swelling and a rapid heartbeat. These are classic symptoms of inflammation and fever, for which cherry has long been indicated. As with many members of the rose family, the cyanogens and flavonoids in black cherry work together to sedate and cool the body. The flavonoids help repair arterial irritability and reduce capillary congestion, which can cause cardiac irregularities and nervous heart palpitations, and the small amount of cyanogens adds to its cooling action. Furthermore, it assists to normalize histamine within the system (a part of the natural immune response) and specifically reduces excessive heat and inflammation due to an aggravated histamine reaction. It is for people that tend to have red, irritated reactions on their skin or where tissues around small cuts develop cherry red borders, indicating an excess of histamine.

American Mahogany

One of black cherry's valuable attributes is its beautiful wood, and by the 1700s it was quickly becoming overharvested. Along with black walnut, it is considered one of our most prized lumbers in North American forests. The exquisite wood is strong and hard, with a fine, compact grain. Often referred to as "American mahogany," it polishes to rich reddish brown or warm, amber-orange hues and often fetches a high price. Much sought after by cabinetmakers since colonial days, it is well suited for fine furniture, cabinet work, veneer, flooring and interior trim, and was used as paneling in elegant rooms of English estates. The wood resists shock and pressure, making it suitable for tool handles, canes and walking sticks, and the best and most expensive stocks for muskets and guns were often made of wild cherry. The wood is also very stable in response to changes in humidity, rendering it useful for weighing apparatus, doors and clocks. As fuel wood, it was used in cook stoves, and the sweet smoke imparted a unique flavour to food.

Folklore

According to Serbian folklore, Vilas were beautiful female creatures, similar to fairies and elves, with long, flowing hair and dressed in white. They lived in the hills and woods, often by cherry trees, passing their time singing and dancing. When traveling through the forest riding seven-year-old stags, they made sounds similar to woodpeckers. They were known to break men's hearts as they flew over (as mentioned by J.K. Rowling in her book *Goblet of Fire*) and were rumoured to take children who were abused by their parents to protect them.

In the Middle Ages, it was customary to give salutations when passing a cherry tree to ensure a bountiful harvest. They were connected with energies of abundance and prosperity, and to dream of a blooming cherry tree meant potential good fortune was coming your way. A wish would be granted if whispered to a flowering cherry. They could also be held in confidence as noted in this rhyme;

We have a secret just we three
The robin and I and
the sweet cherry tree

This tree symbolizes love and beauty, and both the flowers and fruit were frequently noted in literature. Associated with Venus, the blossom, fruit, stone and wood were thought to be powerful tools to draw love's energy. Where apples have more of a sinister side to them, cherries symbolize kindness and life's sweetness, particularly when depicted in European paintings.

When young men went off to war, women would promise to plant a berry bush, such as cherry or highbush cranberry, on their grave should they die. This tradition encouraged birds to come and eat the berries and bring news from home to those lying beneath.

Lessons of Cherry

The flowers of cherry help release sadness and despair by evoking the essence of pure joy and peace. They teach us to value each moment so that life doesn't slip by. The wood conveys earth energy and is very grounding, solid and unwavering. It is used to bring stability into your life and provide insight and intuition to help one overcome many obstacles.

Black Walnut

Juglans nigra

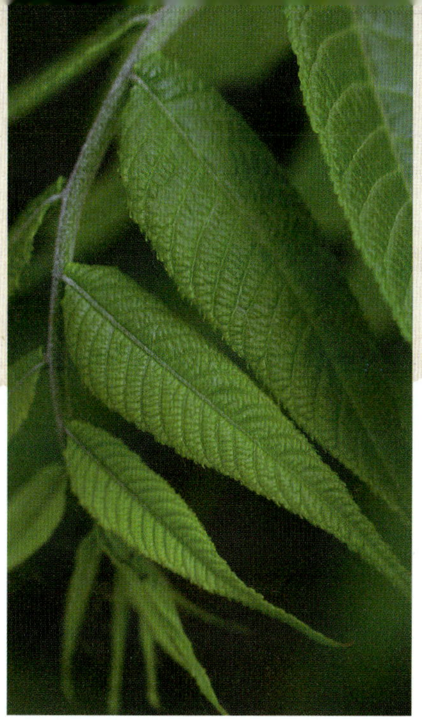

In the corner of our yard, beside the old barn, stands a massive black walnut with strong, spreading branches. Every year, while picking up the nuts off the ground, I breathe in its enchanting scent. This magnificent tree provides many bountiful gifts, and it's an honour to be friends with such a powerful ally.

Black walnuts grow around the Great Lakes, and in Canada only inhabit the very southern regions of Ontario. When the settlers first arrived on these shores, they recorded seeing tall trees in open groves growing abundantly along rivers. These seemingly planted woodlands, which created a park-like setting, were chiefly made up of walnuts. The Indigenous people maintained walnut and oak savannahs by fire, thereby producing ash and open canopies, both essential for good nut production. These open environments also provided homes for other flora and fauna that afforded them additional food.

The Pennsylvania Dutch, who saw groups of black walnuts as an indicator of good soil fertility, settled on lands with healthy stands of walnuts. These trees favour riparian zones, which, due to frequent flooding, offer the deep, rich fertile soils they prefer. Shallow soils are not conducive to walnuts' long tap root, and trees on these sites tend to become stunted and diseased. The deep root serves well to anchor the trees, and wind seldom tips them over. So rarely does one topple that folklore says that a fallen walnut tree is an indication that calamity will soon follow.

Meeting Black Walnut

Black walnuts generally live 150 years but can survive two or three centuries if growing conditions are ideal. They are solitary trees. Being

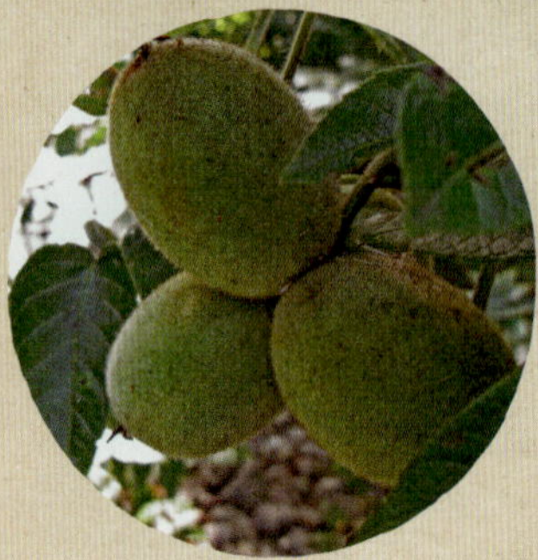

Butternut's elliptical fruit

shade intolerant, they are often one of the first trees to become established when an ecosystem has been disturbed. They flourish in either open savannahs, where they create pure stands, or rich, moist forests with other hardwoods.

Black walnut has a beautiful, graceful appearance. Its long, plume-shaped leaves, which hold 14 to 22 leaflets, gentle droop downwards and when crushed or rubbed release a pleasant, spicy aroma. Its terminal leaflet is either absent or diminished and generally smaller than its lateral counterparts.

Being monoecious, the male and female flowers grow on the same tree and appear in early spring as the leaves emerge. The wind-pollinated flowers soon develop into round fruit with leathery green husks and is the largest nut in northern temperate forests. In contrast, white walnut or butternut's (*Juglans cinerea*) elliptical fruit is covered with dense, sticky hairs. Even though folklore says a large crop of nuts indicates a harsh winter, like many nut trees they generally bear heavy yields every second or third year and need sunlight to do so. Nuts from both species require a season of freezing in the ground before germination.

Walnuts are late to come into leaf in spring, and their golden autumn leaves shed early, leaving its dark, bare skeleton exposed for much of the year. When covered in foliage, it has a delicate, feminine look, but once the leaves fall, silence reigns and the massive, heavy branches give the tree a masculine appearance. In fall and into the winter, the conspicuous nests of the fall webworm (*Hyphantria cunea*) can be seen hanging from the ends of the branches as a ragged mass of silk, and although unsightly, the larvae do not harm otherwise healthy trees.

Juglone Toxicity

One of the few things people seem to know about black walnut is that it is allelopathic. Walnuts are solitary trees, producing their own chemical warfare to maintain their personal space. They release a toxic substance from their roots, nut hulls and decaying leaves known as juglone, which oxidizes in the soil and inhibits the growth of other sensitive plants that dare to grow within its canopy, including their own seedlings. However, if you have seen a nut fall, especially ones from the top of the tree, they often bounce. Nuts that bounce away from their mother may someday become a majestic tree. The exact role of juglone remains unknown, but most agree it is likely to reduce competition from neighbouring plants. Butternuts also secrete this chemical, but to a lesser extent.

Its toxic trait has been well documented for centuries, right back to Pliny the Elder, an early Roman naturalist, who wrote in his book *Historia Naturalis*, "the shadow of the walnut is poison to all plant within its compass, and it kills whatever it touches." At that time, another name for walnut was "root of evil," likely named for its poisonous nature. Although it is an impressive shade tree, many gardeners dislike walnuts, claiming them to be messy and affecting the growth of their plants when situated close to their beds. Indeed, many plants, from tomatoes to pines, are afflicted by "walnut wilt"; however, not all are sensitive. Black raspberries (*Rubus occidentalis*) positively flourish under walnuts, and forage grasses grow well beneath its boughs. In fact, pastures and hay fields are said to improve by planting walnut borders. It seems several native wildflowers, trees and shrubs that have evolved with walnuts are tolerant to juglone, but many alien garden plants that have no evolutionary experience with its allelopathic chemical are sensitive.

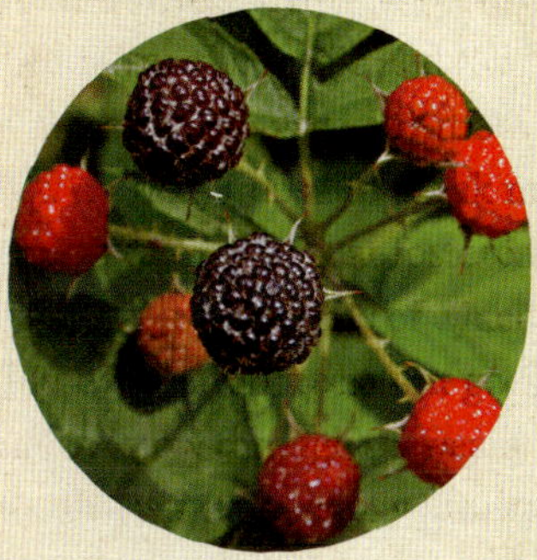

Black raspberry

Walnut's Close Cousins

When I return from our frequent forest walks, I often notice that I have gained a pocket full of hickory nuts. Children gather them along the way and are then handed to me for safekeeping. Some still hold their green husks, while others have teeth marks where grey squirrels have gnawed on them. No matter; they somehow make their way back to the house only to be found next time I reach into my pocket.

Hickories are closely related to

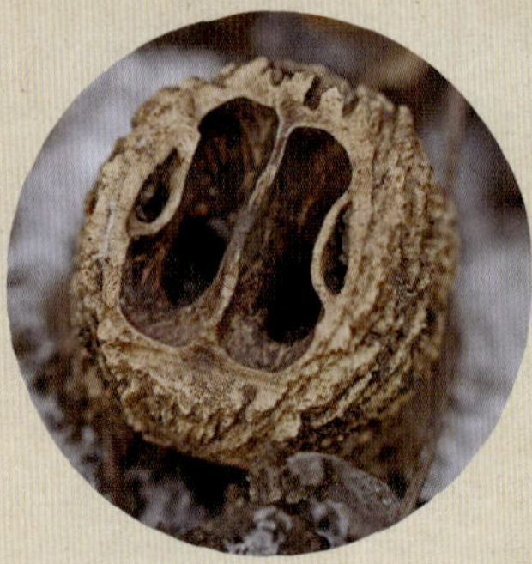
Black walnut eaten by a gray squirrel

walnuts. Most are native to North America, and although we have a variety of species in Southern Ontario, the two most prominent in the landscape are bitternut (*Carya cordiformis*) and shagbark hickory (*Carya ovata*). *Pohickory* is its Algonquin name, derived from pawcohiccora, the term they gave to the milk pressed from the pounded nuts. Pohickory was eventually shortened to give us the name hickory. Bitternut hickory's inedible nut has a loathsome taste and the kernel is so mouth-puckering that only squirrels habitually eat them. These little critters gaily bury the nuts in the fall and are the principal agents of dispersal. Although not eaten by humans, the nuts were commonly collected and pressed into lamp oil, and the wood is said to give ham and bacon the best "hickory-smoked" flavour.

Wildlife Value

Squirrels' adoration of nuts should never be underestimated if you wish to collect some to store. Walnuts are a primary food source for these little critters, and once the nuts fall, they release a chemical that attracts any squirrels in the vicinity. The industrious gray squirrel is the chief harvester of both walnuts and hickories, and their habit of stashing nuts accounts for the distribution of many trees. We draw a great many under our enormous tree as they merrily gather the nuts and hide their buried treasure in our flower beds, only to be discovered in spring when they germinate. We often watch as they boldly sit on their haunches, nibbling away at their snack, while our border collie diligently herds them back up the tree where, in her opinion, squirrels definitely belong. In the woods, the location of walnut trees can be revealed by searching the forest floor for discarded nut shells. Placement of the gnawed opening indicates who has been feeding. Chewing from both sides indicates it has been dined on by a gray squirrel.

As winter approaches, male deer rub against young walnuts to remove the itchy velvet from their antlers, often shredding the bark and leaving it hanging in strips.

This can cause tremendous damage to young saplings but benefits the deer. The rubbing causes the tree to release small amounts of ellagic acid, a compound that helps defend the plant against infections and pests. However, this substance also helps clot blood and can slow bleeding at the antler's stem.

The Nut of the Gods

According to Roman legend, walnut was considered sacred to Jupiter, the mightiest of all gods and ruler of light and sky, as well as thunder, lighting and storms. This speaks volumes about black walnut's powers and gifts. It was alleged that during the "golden age" when man ate acorns, the gods lived on walnuts and thus they became known as "the food of the gods." The botanical name for walnuts was inspired by this idea, and *Juglans* is a contraction of *Jovis glans,* meaning "the nut of Jupiter."

Food Value

Walnuts have been a primary source of nourishment throughout history, providing humanity with high quality fat and protein. They were first mentioned in text dating back 3000 years in ancient Babylon, where they were cultivated for food and noted as a favorite in cuisine. In the eighth century, Charlemagne ordered walnuts to be planted in his extensive orchards, and Medieval cookeries contained numerous recipes featuring walnuts, including a garlic walnut sauce intended for fish. Still popular in the 1800s, walnuts served with Stilton cheese and port became the traditional last course of Victorian upper-class meals.

The best-known walnut for consumption is the English walnut (*Juglans regia*); however, this title is misleading since the tree originated in Persia and has been growing in England only for a few hundred years. Because the nuts are easy to shell, travel well and have a good flavour, it is now the most commonly available walnut in supermarkets.

In North America, black walnuts and butternuts were vital nourishment for the Indigenous people of the Great Lake Region. In 1612, Captain John Smith wrote, "in May and June they planted their fields of corn, beans, squash and tobacco and lived mostly on acorns, walnuts and fish." After settlement, the pioneers quickly learned of their value, and nearly every farm in its range had a nut grove. Although our native walnuts are very delicious, they never enjoyed commercial success because the shells, which are thicker than those of the English walnut, are very difficult to crack, making them unpopular with growers. On the other hand, butternut kernels were recognized for their sweetness and high oil content, ranking them as our most valued nut. Once plentiful in stores, they were highly sought after, but now, because of the tree's decline due to a fungal disease known as Butternut Canker, the nuts are seldom found. Hickory nuts were also commonly gathered but the southerly pecan (*Carya illinoinensis*) is the only hickory commercially grown.

Our native walnuts are a rich source of quality plant-based fat and protein. The oil within the nut is very high in Omega 3 fatty acids and has great antioxidant qualities. Pound for pound, walnuts and beef have equal value of protein, making walnuts an essential food in vegetarian diets. They add a wonderful flavour to baked goods and are tasty in salads. They can be ground into nut butter or pressed into quality vegetable oil, which is highly prized by chefs for its light, delicate flavour.

During the winter months, when food was scarce, the Indigenous peoples ate them raw, roasted, or ground into meal to be added to breads, cakes or soups. Early Canadian inns coated them with sugar or honey and served them to guests. Another favorite recipe was to pickle the young green nuts in their husks and consume them with meat. Like hickory nuts, the Indigenous people pounded walnuts into a fine mash, boiled them in water and skimmed off the oily liquid that swam to the surface to make a sweet "nut milk." This was added to hominy, beans, squash, soups and bread to add nourishment and provide a rich, pleasing taste.

Harvesting the Nuts

It was said that beating the tree would improve the quality of the fruit. This may be due to the fact that using a stick to knock walnuts out of trees was once the main method of harvest so that the better nuts could be obtained. Generally, however, only nuts that drop naturally are ready to husk, since those picked from the tree are too green and refuse to release their nut. The husk surrounding the shell does not split apart like that of hickory nuts. To facilitate their removal, the hulls should be at their dark, spongy stage. Put a piece of one centimeter (half-inch) square mesh hardware cloth on the ground, place a few nuts on it and forcefully slide your boot over the hulls, allowing the rolling action on the mesh to remove the hull from its shell.

Once most of the husks are removed, drop the nuts into a five-gallon bucket of water and agitate them vigorously to help remove any remaining hull. Spread them out in the sun until the shells are thoroughly dry. It is necessary to keep them away from squirrels, for these little critters are cheerfully blatant about their nut-stealing abilities. When the nuts are dry, disperse them thinly and store them in a cool, dark, ventilated place for about four months to cure. This helps to separate the kernel from the shell and allows them to develop their rich, unique flavour.

To crack the nut, wrap it in a clean cloth and hold it vertical on a flat rock or hard surface. Strike the base with a hammer until it breaks, then unwrap it and pick out the loose pieces. Alternatively, you can close a vise on the nut, which damages fewer nut meats. After the nuts are cracked, they can be eaten right away or frozen.

Going Nuts

According to the Medieval Doctrine of Signatures, which attributes the therapeutic properties of a plant based on its similarity to a specific body part, it was reasoned that walnuts were beneficial for mental illnesses because the meat kernel resembled the brain and the shell a human skull. In his book *Adam in Eden,* written in 1657, William Cole wrote, "walnuts have the perfect signature of the head ... the inner woody shell hath the sign of the skull ... and kernel hath the very figure of the brain and therefore it is very profitable for the brain."

Walnuts have long been tied to mental powers, and eating the nut was believed to cure and prevent madness. Science has now shown there is some truth in this. Walnuts are packed with antioxidants and high levels of essential fatty acids that help rebuild and strengthen brain cells. Few foods are as high in these omega 3 fatty acids, which are necessary for healthy brain development in young children. They also assist in maintaining cognitive powers as we age and may help reduce the risk of Alzheimer's disease. One only needs to eat a few each day to reap its benefits. Known as brain food, walnuts at one time were given to people who were showing signs of mental aberration or becoming forgetful. Thus, the term "going nuts" or "off one's nuts" came to mean going crazy and these "nut cases" often ended up in the "nut house."

These benefits have been known since antiquity, and even King Solomon of Israel, who lived a thousand years before Christ and was recognized for his vast wisdom, had orchards of walnuts. He was

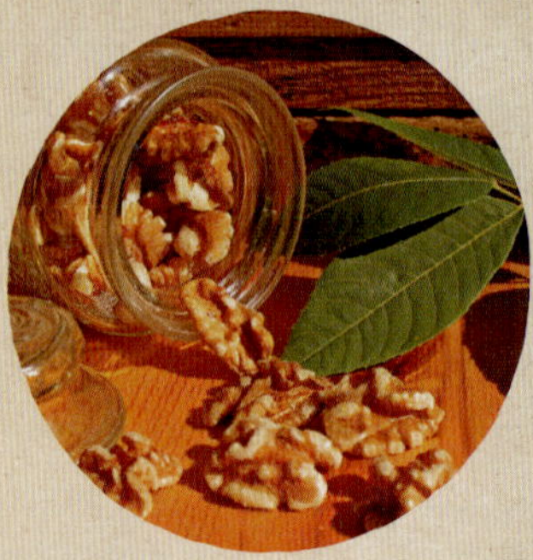

Walnuts are packed with antioxidants and essential fatty acids

said to take short breaks in his groves to eat the nuts, and perhaps this is why he was so wise. Today, walnut trees continue to be a symbol of intelligence, wisdom and knowledge; inspiration, intellect and mental aptitude all come under its realm.

Medicinal Uses

During the nineteenth century, butternut was the preferred member of the family used therapeutically, and most herbal references cited in America refer to this species. Today the roles have reversed and black walnut seems to be the medicine of choice. It appears the two species can be used somewhat interchangeably, and it is the naphthoquinone juglone present in both species that gives them their purgative, antimicrobial and parasite-inhibiting powers.

Butternut is well suited for stimulating the bile and gently purging the intestines and is primarily used for constipation, diarrhea, parasites and skin issues associated with intestinal problems. Black walnut is employed for similar conditions; however, due to the tannic acids in the leaves, it provides additional astringent actions. It also has a subtly toning effect on the cardiovascular system and influences the thyroid.

For medicine, it is the hulls, leaves and bark that are most commonly used. In folk medicine, the black hulls were traditionally employed, but the green unripe husks are recommended by some herbalists. The leaves are gathered in early summer. The bark is collected in spring when the sap is running and dried for more than a year to reduce its purgative and griping properties.

Actions on Digestion

By the eighteenth century, walnut hulls and inner bark had the reputation of being one of the best and safest available purgatives known and a specific for dysentery. In 1817, Jacob Bigelow wrote that "it affords one of the most mild and efficacious laxatives we possess," and Peter Smith (1812) recommended it "in a weak and debilitated state of the bowels." It acts as a safe stimulus and tonic to the system, producing good habits so that constipation and irregularity are removed and the bowels are encouraged to function well and healthy. As herbalist Matthew Wood describes, "The hulls are indicated in constipation, because they purge out impacted bowels; in diarrhea, because they purge out heat and infection; in parasite infection, because they kill low forms of life."

Walnut helps coordinate the digestive tract by increasing digestive secretions and maintaining a steady flow of bile from the gallbladder to ensure healthy function. This helps correct constipation from lack of bile, alleviate a congestion gallbladder, relieve jaundice, aid in the removal of gallstones and flush diarrhea due to bacterial infections. As well as acting on the bowels, walnut has a marked influence upon the skin, especially chronic issues that are connected to disorders of the intestines, liver and gallbladder.

Over time, walnut imparts a desirable toning impression on the mucous membranes and muscles of the intestinal walls. It is used for irritated and inflamed bowels, colic, dysentery and to help prevent the uptake of toxins from congested bowels or a leaky gut. Its ability to tone tissues goes beyond the digestive tract, and walnut also has a remarkable effect on the blood vessels. Thus, it is well suited for prolapsed anuses, ballooned intestines, bleeding hemorrhoids, ruptured arteries and swollen veins.

Cardiovascular System

The leaves have an old reputation for strengthening the heart and vascular system. Because they are toning to the blood vessels, they ultimately supply nutrients to the organs in the body. Walnut may also alleviate venous congestion and remove fatty deposits in the arteries that can lead to arteriosclerosis. On top of this, the essential fatty acids, melatonin and vitamin E found in the nuts helps the nervous system function properly, protects the heart and reduces the risk of heart disease, making them a great addition to a healthy diet.

Thyroids

Healthy thyroids disperse a small amount of iodine throughout the body, and because black walnut contains potassium iodine, it hints at its use as thyroid medication. The hulls were traditionally employed for goiters and they continue to be used as an excellent remedy for hypothyroidism, especially when combined with chickweed. Walnut has proven successful at getting people off thyroid medication, working about 50 percent of the time. Iodine is also essential for breast health, and a deficiency may cause problems such as fibrocystic breast disease and breast cancer; therefore, walnut may benefit these concerns.

It is a remedy that purifies the blood. Toxemia or "bad blood" is often believed to be caused by poor elimination or a faulty liver, but it can also be caused by a deficient metabolism on a cellular level from a low-functioning thyroid. Historic records indicate that black walnut was used for rheumatism and arthritis. Fibromyalgia, a term used today for rheumatism, is a characteristic symptom of those with hypothyroidism.

Parasites and Fungal Diseases

The juglone present in walnuts kills low life forms, including intestinal parasites, and a strong decoction of the hulls and leaves has been traditionally used to expel worms. Moreover, this constituent has pronounced antifungal and antibacterial activities, making it useful for inhibiting a wide variety of microorganisms. A compress made from black walnut husks is a potent inhibitor of skin fungal infections such as impetigo, cradle cap, ringworm and athlete's foot, and is renowned for treating toenail fungus.

Skin Issues

Walnuts contain organic iodine that is more antiseptic and healing to infected cuts and sores than chemical iodine, and its mild hemostatic action helps prevent excessive bleeding. When applied to fresh wounds it slows the flow of blood, discourages infection, prevents swelling and encourages healing. A strong infusion of the husks or leaves applied outwardly makes an excellent curative wash for old sores, ulcers, eczema, acne, abscesses, boils, rashes, shingles and other chronic skin eruptions.

Hair Restorative

The aboriginal people used the extracted oil from the nut in their hair for its restorative abilities. At the same time in Europe, both the green husks and leaves infused in oil were traditionally used because it "stayeth the hair from falling and maketh it fair." This preparation was used for hair loss due to sickness, head parasites or scalp disease and is still found in some natural shampoos, imparting a pleasant, citrusy scent.

As originally described by Pliny in the first century, Roman women used the hulls to darken the silver of aging and enhance their appearance. For centuries, different recipes were used, but walnut remained a main constituent of hair dye until the beginning of the twentieth century.

Valuable Wood

Although gardeners may not appreciate walnut's charms, this is not the case with woodworkers, and there is no more highly valued timber in North America then black walnut. The clear wood sells for an exceptional price and it is not uncommon to net several thousand dollars for a single tree. During the 1700s, carpenters chiefly used walnut, along with black cherry and curled maple, for their craft, and it soon became increasingly rare.

Black walnut wood has a beautiful, lustrous, dark brown colour with occasional streaks of purple, and when viewed or lit from different angles it can change colours. It not only is strong and durable, the heavy, hard wood is naturally resistant to decay, easily worked, has a straight grain and polishes well. This provides the creative entrepreneur opportunities for making fine furniture, cabinet work, tables and chairs, chests of drawers, flooring and wall paneling. It is also fashioned into smaller articles, including pulleys and cogs, knife hilts, and is an excellent candidate for turning wooden bowls. Walnut makes good fuel wood, and the fragrant smoke is likened to tea leaves; however, due to its high value, many feel it is a crime to burn, and in some regions, it was even considered bad luck to do so.

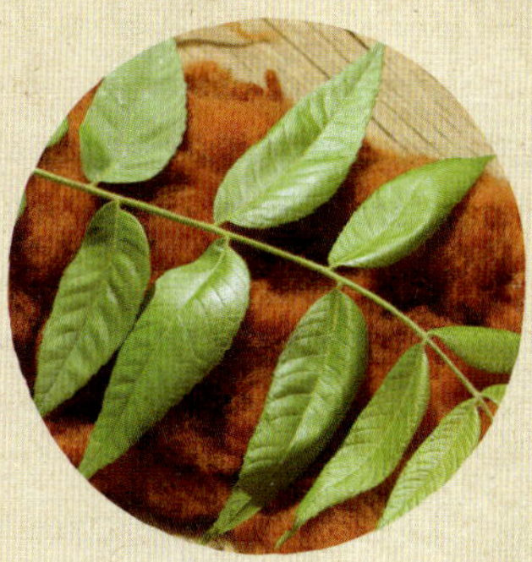

Black walnut dye from hulls

Harder than oak and extremely stable once seasoned, walnut holds its shape well and is not likely to shrink or warp. This made it the wood of choice for gunstocks and some of the finest rifles and guns made flaunt its wood. So common was its use that by the 1820s the expression "to shoulder walnut" meant you were going off to fight.

Source of Natural Dye

The presence of juglone, particularly in the husks, is responsible for producing a brown staining pigment that is useful for artisans.

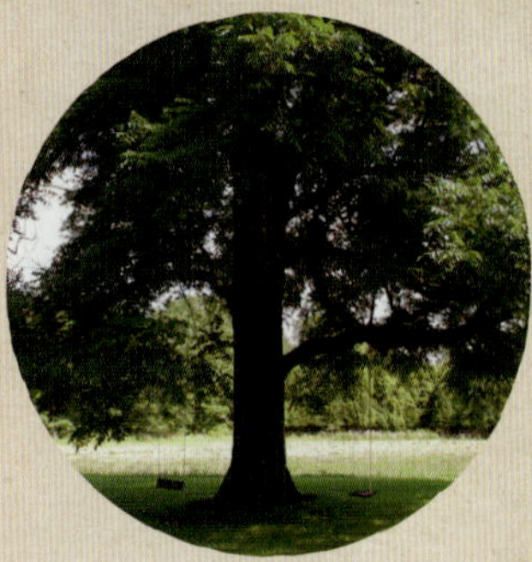

Massive black walnut tree

Anyone who has handled the nuts knows this, and their hands will be stained a dark brown colour that will last for days. Kalm, a botanist who spent three years (1748 to 1751) exploring plants in eastern North America, wrote that the green peel that enclosed the nut "if handled frequently will yield a black colour which cannot be got off the fingers in two- or three-weeks' time, though the hands are washed ever so much. It is therefore not advisable to carry these nuts with their green shells in any cloth, for it will then be spoiled."

Indeed, the hulls produce a first-class caramel-brown dye that has been used for centuries. It is still very popular because the colourant binds directly to the fibres without the assistance of a mordant to hold the dye. It was common practice among colonial women to colour their homespun wool with walnut.

The hulls and inner bark of butternut also yields a permanent dye that coloured homespun clothing various hues of yellows and browns, and when boiled with blue clay would create a deep black shade. Known as the original khaki, it was butternut that coloured the uniforms of Confederate soldiers during the Civil War, and the southern soldiers were often referred to as "butternuts."

Other Uses

Walnut has many other gifts. The kernel yields oil that is useful for finishing wood products, especially items associated with food, such as wooden spoons, salad bowls and bread boards. In nineteenth century, France, walnut oil was used in the church as holy oil, and European artists favoured it as a paint medium to be mixed with pigment. French Impressionists preferred it to linseed oil, and chemical analysis shows that paintings of Monet, Pissarro, and Cezanne carry traces of walnut oil. Scribes made a rich brown or black ink from walnut hulls, and both Leonardo da Vinci and Rembrandt used it in their art.

The finely ground shells serve to polish and clean metal, wood and stone, and are used to clean automobile and jet engines. They are incorporated into winter tires, acting like tiny spikes that dig into ice and snow to provide added traction, and are useful as exfoliates in soaps and face cleaners in the cosmetic industry.

Another characteristic of walnut is that its juglone has the ability to sedate fish. Like hickory husks, the Indigenous people and early pioneers threw the mashed green hulls into pools of water to stun fish and bring them to the surface so that they were easier to catch. According to fishing regulations, this is now an illegal practice in most provinces and states. Incidentally, if you have troubles with the law, burning a piece of hickory root to ashes and placing the ashes in a box over the doorway is believed to keep police at bay.

Home and Garden

As early as the first century, walnut was employed as a deterrent to insect pests. By the seventeenth century, John Evelyn noted that "the very husks and leaves, being macerated in warm water, and that liquor poured on the carpet of walks and bowling greens does infallibly kill the worms, without endangering the grass." Another added advantage to the juglone is its apparent ability to ward off mosquitos and flies. German author and forester Peter Wohlleben wrote, "Walnuts have compounds in their leaves that deal so effectively with insects that garden lovers are often advised to put a bench under a canopy of walnuts if they want a comfortable place to relax in the garden, because this is where they will have the least chance of being bitten by mosquitoes." Farmers planted them around their barns to ward off flies, and the fresh leaves were scattered about homes to discourage insects.

Most likely due to its connection to Jupiter, the god of thunder and lightning, walnut was used for weather magic. There is another curious bit of folklore telling of how to end a drought. When the weather was dry, a piece of walnut bark that had been struck by lightning was placed in a cup of water. Rain, it was said, was ensured within two days. The bark was then dried and saved for future use.

Fertility

On our family farm, our massive black walnut tree has a prominent place by the barn, and I've often wondered if the stately tree was planted years earlier by the original homesteaders or whether an industrious squirrel just forgot where it buried its nut. Since then, older farmers have told me that walnuts were once commonly planted around barnyards to increase the fertility of cattle and encourage more milk production. Perhaps the upsurge in productivity was caused by an improvement of pasture grass or the deterrent of flies that pestered the livestock. On the other hand, to prevent horses from becoming ill, folklore warns not to plant walnuts near stables.

In legends, walnuts were connected to fertility and love. The Romans and Greeks ate the nuts to increase fertility, and during the Medieval period the nut was carried in its shell for the same purpose. Although considered a masculine tree, the Romans also gave walnut a feminine aspect, connecting it to not only Jupiter but also his wife Juno, the goddess of women, fertility, marriage and love. For this reason, the Romans once buried coins beneath walnut trees as an offering to the goddess, and during weddings it was customary to throw walnuts at the bride and groom to promote fertility. Considering their size, this seems like a painful and hazardous practice.

The nuts were also carried to awaken the fertility of the mind, which takes us back to the fact that they build and strengthen the brain.

Folklore

In Italian folklore, walnut trees are linked with witches. It was said that witches preferred to meet under the shade of the walnut and could be seen dancing under their boughs during their sacred rites. For centuries, legends were told of the great witch gathering in the town of Benevento at the site of an ancient walnut tree. In the year 662, the church had the tree removed. The witches of Benevento replanted the tree where the original stood, and it is said that it, or possibly an offspring, still stands in the town. Today, bottles of Strega liqueur made in Benevento still bear labels that display the old walnut tree with a group of witches dancing around it.

Another superstition held that if a walnut was dropped into the lap of a person suspected of casting curses, that person would remain rooted to the spot and unable to rise as long as the nut remained in place.

Perhaps it is the walnut's pungent aroma, the dropping nuts or its complex branches that emit a strong, stimulating energy that makes sleeping difficult beneath it. Thus, in conjunction with these traits, falling asleep under a walnut tree was thought to cause madness. Travelers were warned not to choose walnut trees as a refuge for the night, fearing they might become ill.

Keeping a bowl of walnuts on the table radiates the power of Jupiter and brings new opportunities and wealth to the family within and if someone gives you a bag of walnuts, all your wishes will be fulfilled. People once placed walnut leaves around their head or in their hat to prevent headaches or sunstroke, and it was suggested that carrying a walnut in your pocket could ward off the evils of rheumatism.

Walnuts were also used to "fall out of love" with someone. Bathing in an infusion made with nine walnut leaves and then throwing the water against the tree will renounce any ties to a former lover and expel or remove feelings no longer wanted.

Walnuts are famous for their strong husk and a shell that is hard to crack. Throughout history, the shells were often used as containers to hide magical or precious objects. In Hans Christian Andersen's fairytale, Thumbelina slept in a beautifully polished walnut shell, and due to his tiny size, Tom Thumb also lived inside one. The long tradition of hiding things and keeping them safe within the hard case speaks to the protective qualities of walnuts.

Lessons of Black Walnut

To be titled the "nut of the gods" speaks volumes of the walnut's sacred powers and gifts. This is a tree that likes to be on its own, growing where the sun shines and defending the land on which it stands. Sitting under its boughs gives you a sense of independence. It is for those who are too much under the influence or domination of others and have a fear of choosing their own unique path in life. It gives us the strength to take charge and make the changes needed to become more independent. It teaches us to accept and honour who we are and encourages us to appreciate others as individuals.

As reflected by its protective shell, it provides protection from outside influences that prevent us from growing to our full potential. Along with these protective attributes, it also has strong expelling qualities, as seen in its very nature of producing juglone. This allelopathic property provides fortification in ridding oneself of unwanted habits or emotions such as sadness, grief or other negative feelings. It is for those navigating through times of challenge and loss and Matthew Wood suggests it is for both adults and children going through a bad divorce, allowing them to get beyond the experience.

As a tree that produces nuts that strengthen the brain, walnut can help us use our mental gifts more wisely. Where the beech tree is symbolic of ancestral wisdom, walnut represents mental wisdom. It teaches us clarity and focus, and communicates how to best use our intelligence. This allows us to clearly distinguish between illusion and reality, so that we become more aware of our surroundings, and reminds us to use discernment to better understand a situation before making a decision.

Elderberry

Sambucus canadensis

Black Elderberry, Common Elder, Canadian Elder, American Elder, Black-Berried Elder, Sweet Elderberry, Elder Blow, Ellum Blow Tree, Elder Blossom Tree, Lady Elder, Bore Tree, Bour Tree, Pipe Tree and Hylder

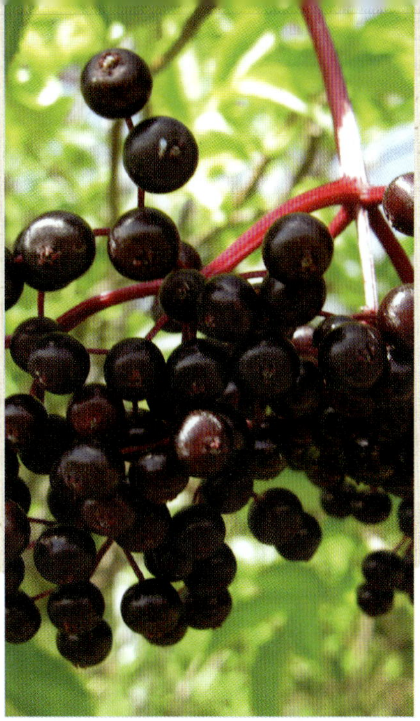

Grandmother elder has a strong, yet compassionate spirit. It is believed she descended from the stars as a teacher and healer to all those on earth. She is beloved by those who know her, and the old Austrian saying, "Tip your hat to the elder," indicated that people throughout history held her in high regard. To this day, many still pay homage when passing, with a quick doff of the cap or a nod of the head, to acknowledge her many gifts, and each spring, offerings are placed at her roots in hopes of a good crop and healing medicine.

Meeting Elder

European black elderberry (*Sambucus nigra*) is considered a small tree and is somewhat larger than our Canadian elderberry (*Sambucus canadensis*), which generally only reaches heights of three meters. They tolerate some shade, but grow faster and produce more flowers and fruit in sunny locations. They propagate easily from cuttings and a twig poked in the ground will likely take root. This trait made elder an ancient symbol of death and regeneration.

In early summer, the shrub is covered with creamy-white, flat-topped blossoms that bob and sway in the breeze. They are particularly attractive shimmering in the sunlight or when the morning dew settles lightly upon them. The airy umbels contain hundreds of tiny florets, each with five petals and an enchanting fragrance. They are followed by dark, purple berries attached to red stems that hang

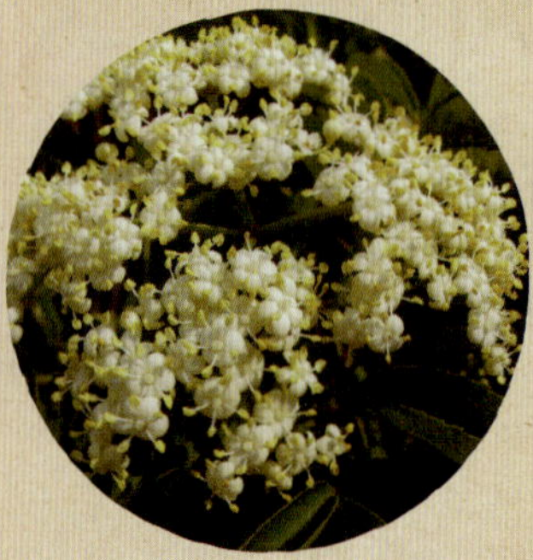

Elder's creamy white blossoms

in dense clusters. The fruit ripen in late summer and are heavy with juice, drawing in hordes of birds before fall migration. The leaves, flowers and fruit are thought to represent the three phases of the Goddess: maiden, mother and hag, respectively. The Celts also believed the elder marked the progression of the seasons. The leaves emerge early and herald the return of spring. The sweetly scented blossoms arrive around midsummer, commencing the upcoming growing season. When the berries are fully ripe, summer is coming to an end, signifying darkness will soon follow. As the leaves change colour and fall from their branches, winter begins, and it is then that elder's medicinal gifts are truly treasured.

In the Garden

The deep green leaves create a nice backdrop in large gardens and provides effective shelter from the elements. *The Mystery of Husbandry,* written in 1697 by John Worlidge, noted that elderberry was "necessary and proper for fencing and enclosing of lands." It went on to say that elders provided "speedy shelter for a garden from winds, beasts and such like injuries and from rude michers (a lurking thief or skulking vagabond)." It was rumoured to benefit a variety of garden plants because it served as a tutelary spirit or guide for others. Lady Elder also appeases the fairies, as the wee folk are most likely to swing and play in such trees.

Wildlife Value

The bisexual flowers produce highly volatile chemicals that attract large numbers of tiny beneficial insects, but because little nectar is produced, most visitors are pollen feeders. They are not commonly visited by bees and wasps, making small flies, gnats, midges and beetles responsible for the majority of pollination.

The pith inside the young branches is soft and as the branches age, the wood thickens and the pith disappears. The hollow stems make useful nesting chambers for wild bees and spiders. They are also used by a small potter wasp that partitions off larva cells and stocks them with paralyzed caterpillars and other insects. An egg is then laid in each cell and sealed with mud. After the young hatch they consume the insect, providing them easy access to food.

Because elderberries provide vast amounts of fruit that are consumed by birds and mammals, biologists often plant them in natural areas to restore wildlife habitat. More than 40 bird species eat the berries and are the chief distributors of the seeds. This is observed by the number of shrubs that spring up around fence posts and other similar perches where seeds have been deposited through bird droppings. Elderberries are valued by fall migratory birds, fueling up for the trip south. Squirrels, chipmunks, mice, rabbits, raccoons, foxes, opossums and bears also enjoy the fruit, while catbirds and indigo buntings frequently construct their nests in the branches, making them their home.

Meaning of its Name

The name elder may be traced to the Anglo-Saxon word *aeld*, meaning fire, and indicates that the hollow stems were used to blow on newly kindled fires to increase the flames. In Iceland, the faeries are still taken very seriously and are known as the *huldafolk*, or hidden people. Thus, the name elder may have instead originated from hulda, suggesting that faeries frequent the small trees.

The generic name *sambucus* appears in the literature of Pliny and other early writers, and was derived from the Greek word *sambuca* or *sambuke*, an ancient musical instrument. Because elder's hard branches polish readily and the soft pithy core is easily removed, a woodwind instrument or a pan pipe was made from the hollowed-out stems, known as a sambuca. Italian peasants and shepherds also constructed simple flutes suitable for making music, called sampogna.

As everyone knows, elves and fairies love music, dancing and merrymaking. Because instruments made from elder wood make the most haunting sounds, flutes, whistles, chanters or pipes constructed from this tree are said to produce the music fairies love best. They were employed to call in these earth spirits, as they were readily drawn to the source, and the Druids used them to communicate with the souls of the dead.

Cyanide Poisoning

This small tree contains small amounts of cyanide-producing glycosides called sambunigrin. It is found in the leaves, bark, roots, unripe fruit and seeds, and can be toxic if eaten in sufficient quantities. When the leaves are crushed, sambunigrin gases are released into the air, giving the plant its unique smell. Eating large measures of the uncooked berries may cause an emetic effect, producing symptoms of nausea, vomiting and diarrhea. Therefore, due to the mild cyanide content, it is recommended to cook or dry the berries before consumption, as this destroys the glycoside compounds.

Culinary Uses

The Indigenous people made pemmican using dried elderberries, dried meat and fat to provide nourishment through the winter months. The deep purple berries are loaded with antioxidants and contain high levels of vitamin C, as well as vitamin A, iron, calcium and potassium. For easy winter storage, freeze the berries and used in pancakes, pies, muffins or cakes.

The ripe berries make a delicious cold drink that is popular with children. To make, simmer the mashed berries for fifteen minutes with a small amount of water, then strain out the liquid through some cheesecloth. After adding sweetener, dilute it with other fruit juices or mix it with carbonated water for a sparkling beverage. Elderflowers soaked in water and lemon juice overnight also provide a refreshing summer drink. The berries are extensively used in red wines, ports, cordials and other liqueurs for colouring and flavouring, and delicate wines and champagnes are made from the flowers. Elderberry wine served at Samhain (Halloween) is considered a sacred gift bestowed on us from Mother Earth.

The frothy creamy-white flowers, soaked in brandy for ten minutes, then dipped in batter and fried, make delicious fritters when served with maple or elderberry syrup. As well, adding the flowers to cakes and muffins provides a delicate texture. For centuries, the delicious fruit have been used in relish, chutney and ketchup recipes, and today they are included in meat sauces, syrups, fruit rolls, pies and tarts. The berries have little natural pectin, so commercial pectin must be added when making jellies and jams. In Japan, elderberries are still used as a natural food colouring.

Medicinal Uses

Black elder (Sambucus nigra) is held in highest regard in European tradition, whereas the Canadian elder (Sambucus canadensis) is the remedy of choice in North America. The two are used interchangeably and are so widely employed in folk medicine that elder is described as "an entire pharmacopoeia in one plant." It was a staple remedy in both Europe and North America and frequently designated as "the medicine chest of the country people." In the past it was credited as being a cure for essentially all known illnesses, and in 1664, gardener and herbalist John Evelyn wrote, "if the medicinal properties of its leaves, bark, berries and flowers were thoroughly known, I cannot tell what our countrymen could ail for, which he might not fetch a remedy from every hedge, either for sickness or wounds." As it was used continuously since antiquity, ancient physicians and scholars, including Hippocrates and Pliny the Elder, considered it a great healer and employed it "to cure every ill that flesh is heir to." This useful herb was often included in monastery gardens, and even Charlemagne (800 AD) ordered that an elderberry be planted in every garden in his realm to be a "medicine cabinet ready for immediate use."

Traditionally, every part of the plant has been used as medicine at one time or another, but it is the berries and flowers that are most commonly used today. When taken internally, they are the safest and reflect the overall properties of the plant. Due to their strong purgative action, the leaves are recommended for external use only, as an ointment or poultice. Traditionally, the blooms were picked in the moonlight when they were as "full as your fingers" (the size of one's hand) and the berries gathered when they were dark purple and full of juice. When dry, the flowers turn a dingy brownish-yellow colour and are made into infusions. The fresh flowers can be tinctured, and the berries are most often made into delicious syrup. Energetically, elderberry is cooling and drying, and when properly prepared the flowers and ripe berries are quite safe and effectual. Benefiting both the beginning and end of life, it is used for infants and the elderly alike.

Tonic for Longevity

In the seventeenth century, John Evelyn wrote that an extract of the berries "assists longevity," and it was habitual for the British to drink elderberry wine as a way to prolong their life. In the Celtic culture, elderberry tonic was given to the old and sick to protect the heart and keep their bones healthy and strong. Now found to be high in antioxidants, this herb helps counteract cell destruction caused by toxic molecules known as free radicals, and reverses cell damage associated with aging. It is considered an aid for aging eyes and to help adjust the sight from varying light levels, and its blood building abilities help combat anemia. Today, it can be of assistance in detoxification programs by helping rid the body of drugs and cigarette smoke.

Valuable for Fevers

Hans Christian Andersen incorporated elder into his fairy tales. In one of his stories, a young boy was out playing in a puddle on a rainy day. In the evening, his mother gave him a cup of elder blossom tea and sent him to bed. The boy soon fell into a dream where the "Little Elder Mother" took him faraway on a journey to the south. When he awoke, he told his mother that it was hot in this land. Seeing the perspiration on his skin, she agreed and was pleased that the herbal tea had been effective.

Fever-reducing herbs, including catnip, peppermint, yarrow and elderflower, help cool the body by promoting sweating. The diaphoretic actions of elder are well known, and this herb excels as a fever remedy. Drinking a hot flower tea encourages a cleansing sweat, and it is one of the first herbs to reach for to drive out a fever and combat cold and flu symptoms. A rob (syrup) made from the berries also encourages perspiration, but with weaker results. Both the flowers and berries contain viburnic acid, which gently encourages the capillaries to open, increases circulation and brings blood to the surface. This helps to dispel excess heat from the center core, release fluids through the pores and cool the body. Elder is considered both a stimulating and sedative diaphoretic, which has a regulating effect on the fever mechanism, and can either bring on perspiration or check sweating. It is suitable for both children and adults alike and given freely for almost every form of fever.

Respiratory Ailments

Traditionally, elderberry syrup or a flower infusion was used for coughs, colds, influenza and other feverish conditions. As an ancient remedy for opening the lungs, combined with its ability to promote perspiration and increase urination, it was particularly useful for preventing and treating respiratory ailments.

Today, studies have demonstrated that elderberry has antiviral and immune-enhancing properties that aid the body in fighting infections. Viruses invade the body by hijacking cells and reprograming them to make more viruses. Research has revealed that a compound present in elderberries, known as hemagglutinin protein, may help break down the enzyme that viruses use to penetrate healthy cells, thereby substantially reducing its ability to replicate. This can help avert or shorten a cold or flu if taken at the first signs of infection. On top of this, elderberry's ability to elevate body temperature encourages immune function and makes it harder for many viruses and bacteria to become established. Studies have shown that those who used Sambucol, an elderberry product widely marketed in Europe as a cold and flu remedy, reduced the length and severity of infection. Furthering its antiviral and immune enhancing capabilities, the berries may also help prevent or shorten the duration of a herpes outbreak and increase resistance to other viral invaders such as chicken pox, measles and possibly West Nile Virus. The berries benefit lower respiratory infections and chest congestion with restricted breathing. Rob of elderberry, where the juice is boiled down with sugar to the consistency of honey, is invaluable for colds, spasmodic coughs, sore throats, bronchitis and asthma.

In pantries, the flowers were once hung in paper bags to dry, and it was said that every good mother would have some on hand to assist her children through winter sicknesses and the aches and pains associated with them. While boosting a healthy fever to kill invading microbes, elderflowers also help break up and clear out excess phlegm that is linked with colds, coughs and influenza. Moreover, it has added benefits of reducing histamine responses, thus easing cold, flu and allergy symptoms. The flowers are commonly used for upper respiratory tract infections and should be considered when clearing congested sinus or relieving a stuffy nose, watery eyes and painful ears. They are classified as astringent and somewhat drying, yet have a subtle moistening and anti-inflammatory effect on the mucous membranes. A traditional remedy for colds and fevers is a tea combining elderflowers, yarrow and peppermint. Before going to bed, drink the tea while bathing in ginger, cayenne and yarrow flowers.

Clears the Channels

Elder's hollow branches are a signature showing its affinity to the tubes of the body, particularly the blood vessels and skin pores. Elderberry opens all the channels. It encourages elimination through urination and perspiration, breaks up catarrh to clear the lungs, gently purges the bowels, and stimulates circulation of the blood and lymph.

The berries serve to promote digestive activities and support liver function. They enhance digestion by moving materials through efficiently to alleviate congestion, stagnation, heat and toxicity in the digestive tract. It also influences the urinary system. Like most diaphoretics, when elder is taken as a cool tea, its diuretic effects are more pronounced. It acts on the kidneys, correcting renal issues and eliminating excess water by encouraging a healthy flow of urine.

By opening the pores and stirring up the blood, it brings fluids to the surface, thereby removing heat, congestion and toxins. Its ability to detoxify the blood makes it useful for skin problems and inflamed rheumatic conditions caused by "humours" getting stuck in the joints. In the late 1800s, an American sailor informed a physician of Prague that getting drunk on dark-red port was a certain cure for rheumatic pains. This observation started a series of studies ending in the discovery that while genuine port wine produced little benefits, the cheap version, adulterated with elderberry juice, often effectively banishes the pain of arthritis, sciatica and other forms of neuralgia.

At one time, premature infants were sponge-bathed in lukewarm elder blossom infusion as a gentle skin tonic and to help open their tubes and pores. The herb not only strengthened the capillaries, thereby aiding the baby's peripheral circulation, it also helped improve their respiration, digestion and kidney function.

Leaf Ointment

In ancient Rome, Hippocrates endorsed elder to promote vomiting and purging. The leaves and bark are strongly emetic and purgative, but in today standards they are generally not recommended for internal use. However, occasionally the fresh, young leaves are made into a poultice, ointment or simple oil to be applied externally. It effectively removes heat and inflammation, and helps break up congealed blood. This cooling remedy treats all kinds of tumors, swellings, sprains, burns, boils, bumps, bruises and other such injuries by dispersing heat and regulating blood flow to speed healing. It is also an old preparation for easing muscle soreness, rheumatic pain, joint stiffness and hemorrhoids. The leaves can be heated in linseed oil until they become crisp, or alternatively, they are steeped in olive oil for six weeks and strained.

Skin Issues

Similarly, a compress of elderflowers is an advantageous treatment to soothe and cleanse cuts, wounds, obstinate sores, ulcers, abscesses and other infectious or inflamed skin conditions. Additionally, a cold flower infusion is applied to sore, inflamed eyes or to take the heat out of burns. Like the leaves, they have the ability to remove stagnation and toxins in the blood, effectively treating bruises and boils. And because they promote sweating by gently dilating the pores, they are highly regarded for itchy rashes, rosacea, eczema or psoriasis.

Cosmetic Uses

At one time, women washed their faces in dew gathered from elderflower to enhance and preserve their youthfulness. Since antiquity, Elderflower Water has been employed as a beauty product for cleansing and improving the skin, and it continues to be valued for its rejuvenating and revitalizing properties. This product was once a common household item, and from the 1600s until Victorian times, every lady kept some in their dressing chamber to ensure a fair complexion. Although it fell out of favour for a number of years, it has recently regained popularity and is once again found in commercial eye lotions and skin cleansers. It still maintains its reputation for effectively keeping the skin fair and white, and free from freckles, aging spots and blemishes.

Elderflowers have many uses, but they particularly shine in two areas: for fevers and to promote healthy skin. It is not uncommon that herbs acting as relaxing diaphoretics also support skin health. Applied to the skin and eyes, it has a mild astringent and emollient effect, which tones, cleanses and softens tissue, and gently stimulates circulation to bring blood and nourishment to the capillaries. This makes it useful for aging skin and reducing wrinkles.

The flowers are also used in hair rinses to bring out natural highlights and to keep hair healthy and shiny. As well, in his *Complete Herbal*, Nicholas Culpeper noted, "the hair of the head washed with the berries boiled in wine is made black." This was referring to the Romans, who used the dark juice from the berries as a hair dye for graying hair.

Insect Repellant

The leaves exude an unpleasant odour when crushed or bruised, making them an effective insect repellent. Bunches of leaves were suspended around gardens, houses, livestock barns and outhouses to discourage insects, and while working the fields, it was common practice to attach elder leaves to horse harnesses to ward off flies.

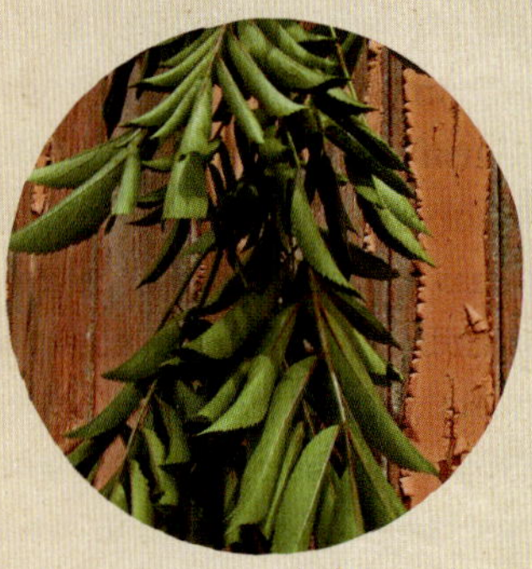

Leaves were suspended around houses, barns and outhouses to discourage flies

Elders were traditionally planted around dairies because they were thought to be effectual in keeping milk from "turning." Cheesecloth used in dairying was hung to dry on elder branches, believing the smell from the leaves contributed to hygiene. Elders were also planted next to bake houses and near kitchens to prevent the devil and other negative influences from being folded into the dough. This folklore may have come from the need to keep flies, and the diseases they carried, away from the food. The custom of cutting a cross on top of the loaf before baking may have stemmed from the same belief. Once baked, loaves and cakes were put out under elderberry bushes to cool, and any food left under them overnight was considered a gift to the fairies.

A Dye Plant

The bark, roots, leaves and berries were all used to manufacture dyes, and elder became an important commodity to the Harris Tweed Company. The bark produced black and grey dyes, the leaves with alum showed yellow-green tones, and the berries with alum generated crimson, blue and purple hues. This historical company still operates today, although it is unlikely they continue to use elder to dye their material.

Popguns, Spigots and Magic Wands

Herbalist and botanist Nicholas Culpeper (1616-1654) made frequent reference to elder in his writings and noted that it was such a common part of society that its portrayal was redundant. He wrote, "I hold it needless to write any description of this, since every boy that plays with pop-guns will not mistake another tree instead of elder." Pliny's text of the first century also verifies that simple instruments, whistle and blow guns were made from this plant.

The soft, white pith in the young stems is easily punched out, leaving a hollow tube that is ideal for making water squirt guns, peashooters and blowguns, and these toys have been fashioned by generations of children.

In addition, there are a number of other uses for elder branches. Hollow sections of the stems were often employed as spindles for weaving and in North America were formed into spiels, known as "elder quills," to tap maple trees for the sap. Beads worn for protection or a talisman to the elder spirit were made by sanding and scraping the bark from young branches and cutting them into bead size pieces to be threaded unto string. As noted in the *Harry Potter* novels, elder held powerful magic when fashioned into wands, and in parts of Ireland, it was rumoured that witches rode brooms made of elder sticks.

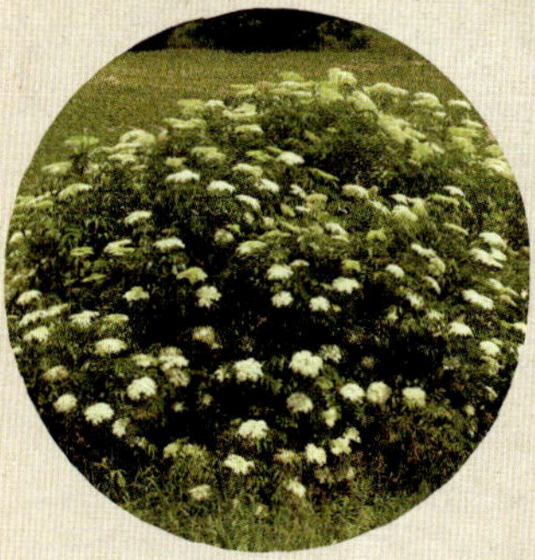

Elder was considered to have protective attributes

Protection

As a result of Elder Mother's compassion for humanity, there has been much folklore written regarding elderberry's protective qualities. Its ability to successfully release enchantments was one of elder's powerful attributes, and it was the tree most often used to undo spells of evil intent. A small, equal-arm cross created from the branches, could be affixed to doors and windows to bring protection against evil influences or to disappoint the "charms of witches." These demons were most often in the form of sickness, many of which Elder Mother could effectively cure.

In common with other trees with white blossoms, such as hawthorn and rowan, it was considered auspicious to have one growing near your house, especially if it seeded there itself. If the rowan's place was traditionally at the front of the house, the elder's station was at the back door, keeping evil from entering the home. If treated respectfully, it blessed those who cared for her, and almost every garden boasted an elder. When this tree had chosen to grow in your yard, it indicated that the Elder Mother had elected to protect your home and farm from lightning and drive away thieves. Growing near cow sheds and stables, it kept livestock from harm and promoted their fertility (possibly due to its ability to repel flies and other insects); therefore, farmers welcomed them on their homesteads.

Death and Regeneration

Elder Mother guarded the entrance to the underworld. She was believed to have the ability to bridge the divide and offer protection for those on their journey to the other side. Archeological findings have confirmed that elder wood was used in funerary rites and crosses of elder were placed on coffins in hopes it would bring peace to the departed. During the spring, elder cuttings were also planted by grave sites. If the branches grew, it indicated that the soul of the person lying beneath was content and had moved on. Luckily, elder propagate well from cuttings.

Blessings

To bless a person, place or thing, elderflower water was sprinkled to the four directions while saying its name. In Victorian times, it was common belief that elder had the power to bring about a marriage. A couple would wed within the year if they were to share a drink of ale infused with elderflowers from the same cup. Elder brought good luck to newlyweds, and if a pregnant woman kissed an elder, it would bless the baby she was carrying.

Christian Mythology

During the rise of Christianity, the church began to oppress any form of tree worship, and because elder was so revered in pagan cultures, it took on negative associations. This beautiful tree became linked with both Judas and Christ's crucifixion and feared in Christian mythology. Judas, so full of remorse for having betrayed Jesus, was believed to have hanged himself from an elder branch. The idea that this bush was chosen is puzzling considering its size and the fact that this modest tree is easily broken. The wood for which the holy cross was made was also believed to be of elder wood and therefore it was portrayed as a tree of sorrow and death. However, according to legend, the elder once grew much taller and only became a stunted and twisted bush as a result of carrying the weight of guilt and remorse. This belief is noted in a verse found in Robert Chambers' *Popular Rhymes of Scotland* (1847):

Bour tree, bour tree crooked rung
Never straight and never strong
Ever bush and never tree
Since our Lord was nailed to thee

Association with Fairies

The elder is endowed with a heavy, somewhat narcotic smell, and Shakespeare called it "the stinking elder." It was considered perilous to nod off under its boughs, and there was a saying, "He who goes to sleep under an Elder-tree will never awaken." Being in its shade is reputed to have a mild influence on the mind and senses, and its slight psycho-active power likely contributed to the many mysterious customs associated with it. In full bloom, the fragrance was believed to put you in a trance or cause giddiness, and many tales have been told of those having visions of the fairy folk as a result of inhaling its aroma. Care was essential, for in Irish folklore, if one fell asleep under the elder you could be whisked away to the fairy realm.

The wee folk might, from time to time, venture into our world, especially on Midsummer Eve. Sitting beneath an elder tree at midnight on the Summer Solstice, particularly when drinking ample quantities of elderflower champagne, would enable you to see the Fairy King and his entire entourage ride by on their way to their Midsummer feast. Under elder's thick canopy, the soothing, relaxing smell could help open your spiritual mind to understand and communicate with these nature spirits and connect you to the natural world around you.

Holes in the countryside where it is easy to enter into fairyland are often found where hawthorns and elders grow. Wood sprites are said to live in elder trees, and when the wind blows through the ellum blows (elder blossoms), it is then that they are riding the branches. These hidden people are companions for children, who often commune and play with them.

The Little Elder Mother

Elder is steeped in folklore and superstition and holds a place of honour and respect in pagan traditions. In Northern Europe, it is associated with a powerful matriarchal dryad or tree spirit, known as the "Little Elder Mother," who dwells in the tree and closely watches over it. For the Druids, this spirit was the goddess of vegetation and presided over the cycle of the seasons, reflecting birth, fruition, death and regeneration. Therefore, the elder tree represents the 13th moon (a short, three-day period over Halloween) in the Celtic Ogham calendar, which ends the agricultural year and begins a new one at Samhain. This is a time of death, but it is also associated with new life, bringing a message of transformation, change and spiritual renewal. This goddess was also considered the guardian of the underworld and presided over the fairy realm. Thus, the elder is thought to serve as a doorway to travel through and connect us with the wisdom of our ancestors.

Like willow, elder has strong feminine associations. Powerful indeed are her blessings, for she is considered to harbor ancient wisdom. It was often called the "witch's tree," and undoubtedly the village hedge witch or herbalist would have used it extensively as medicine and for its healing magic. It was alleged that witches often congregated under both the hawthorn and elder where they were protected in the tree's aura.

Kindling fires with its wood was believed to annoy Elder Mother. This lore may have arisen from the fact that elder makes poor fuel, for the structure of the wood and its sap causes a great deal of spitting, hissing and crackling while burning. To this day, there are those who refuse to burn the dryad's tree in fear of being pursued by misfortune or bad luck. In England, it is believed that to burn elder in your hearth "brings the old lad (the devil) to sit upon your chimney" and food cooked over an elder fire was considered unfit to eat. Others believed that the souls of the dead harbored in the branches; therefore, the wood was never burned for fear they would be lost forever.

It was also imagined that Elder Mother would punish those who harmed her host tree in other ways. It was unwise to cut down or use the tree improperly or with selfish intent, for fear of upsetting her. For this reason, no household furniture was made of elder wood and it was rumoured that babies in elder cradles would get no rest. If you wanted to receive her gifts for rituals, medicine or food, it was appropriate to seek permission before harvesting. Traditionally, this often involved making an offering to the tree and reciting the following rhyme:

Mother Elder, Mother Elder
Give me of thy wood
And I will give thee of mine
When I become a tree

On one hand, Elder Mother was valued for her protective and healing qualities. She was believed to have a benevolent spirit when treated with respect and would generously offer her gifts and blessings to those who protected and cared for the elder tree. On the other hand, elder was feared and became a tree of evil, holding malevolent spirits. These legends were perhaps a way to protect the valued medicine held within the tree. If the tree was cut or burned, the village would lose their medicine and become sick, and to fall ill was considered your misfortune. However, if the tree was treated with deep respect and harvested honourably, in return, it would heal and feed the people for many years. This is an important lesson to learn. It is essential to approach the tree with gratitude and thanks, ask for permission before harvesting and listen with an open heart. Don't harvest if you get a strong intuition not to and be sure to express your deepest appreciation each time you receive her gifts.

Lessons of Elderberry

Elder provides protection and strength to the soul. Her outer wood is strong and hard, offering fortification to the soft inner core where the spirit dwells. She is the gateway guardian; the threshold of consciousness and inner mysteries. Bringing messages of transformation, change and spiritual renewal, she helps increase your awareness so that you can be fully present in the moment to see the "big picture." When you feel stuck in a situation, she awakens you to greater perspectives and better possibilities. With her assistance, your path is always under your feet.

If you open your heart to her, she will gentle guide you through life transformations and bumps in the road, setting your life back on track and reconnecting you to the unity of all life on earth. She helps settle the spirit and promotes feelings of self-worth. Like the woodwind instruments constructed from her branches, she brings sweet music to your ears.

The root of her name is from *aeld*, meaning fire; and she is a lot like fire. Honouring and carefully tending fire makes it a powerful ally, warming your house and cooking your meals. But fire can destroy anything in its path if respect is not granted. So, use her wisely when seeking her guidance, for she has much to teach and offer.

Elm

Ulmus americana and Ulmus rubra (formerly Ulmus fulva)

Ulmus americana

White Elm, American Elm, Water Elm, and Piss Elm

Ulmus rubra

Slippery Elm, Red Elm, Moose Elm and Salve Bark

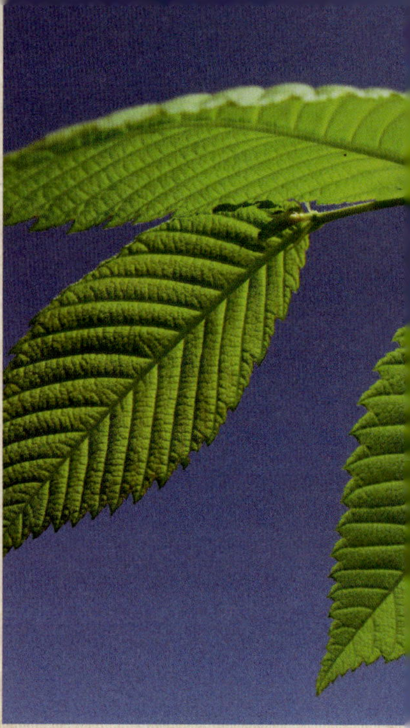

For centuries, the elm tree has been honoured and revered, with its stories being passed down through the generations. In Greek mythology, Orpheus, after rescuing his wife Eurydice from death, paused to play her a love song on his harp. His music was so enchanting that all the animals in the forest gathered around and even the wind stopped to listen. It was said that the first grove of elm sprang out of the earth at this spot.

Street Trees Full of Good Spirits

White elm is well known for its graceful, umbrella-like crown of drooping branches, and from a distance, it is one of the most easily recognized trees. This majestic specimen is thought to be full of good spirits, and its calming energy could be felt by those standing beneath. It was once widely planted in parks and along residential avenues for its stately appearance, and every town seemed to have an Elm Street. Colonists quickly recognized they made good shade trees due to their spreading crowns, fast growth, strong wood and ability to flourish in the relatively poor soils common in urban environments. Their popularity peaked in the years following the American Civil War, and they continued to dominate many village greens, town squares and main streets until they met their demise from the Dutch

Elm Disease in the middle of the twentieth century.

Their spreading canopy held an atmosphere of elegance, and at maturity they formed green, cathedral-like arches that gave a peaceful ambiance to towns. While sitting under an elm tree, nineteenth century American poet Walt Whitman believed it had the ability to inspire pleasant and harmonious thoughts. This metaphor was not recently conceived, for as far back as third century BC, elm trees symbolized an idyllic pastoral life, and their shade created cool, peaceful sanctuaries for both mortals and gods.

The Tree of Justice, Trust and Honesty

Throughout history, people have believed that trees play an important role in society, each with a specific trait. Elms were known as the tree of justice, trust and honesty. During the Middle Ages they were often planted in places where rent and other fees were paid, and as late as the nineteenth century they could be found in public squares near courthouses. Their presence was thought to bring a favourable ruling in court and ensured justice was served. Judges would often pronounce from beneath elms so that the public could be certain their words were honest and trustworthy.

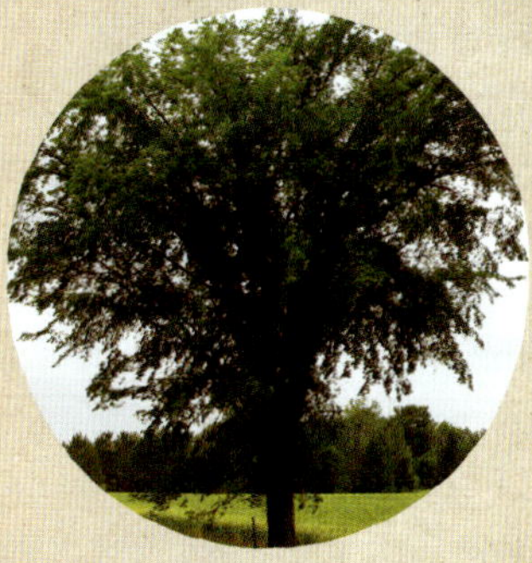

Elms were thought to be full of good spirits

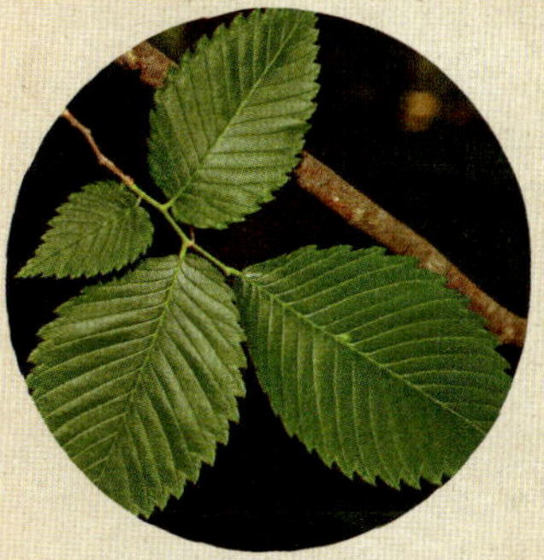

Serrated leaf edges

Meeting Elm

In the *Language of Flowers*, elm denotes dignity and grace, and just by observing its features one can see this comparison is well fitting. It can grow to giant proportions, brushing the sky at 35 meters (120 feet). Before Dutch Elm Disease swept through North America, they made excellent landmark and boundary trees, and it wasn't uncommon to see massive individual specimens lining agricultural fields and roadsides in the rural landscape.

When looking at the leaves, there are two main features that make them easily distinguishable. Frist, the serrated edges comprise unequal teeth, and secondly, they have a lopsided base, where one side of the leaf blade extends farther down the petiole than the other. The foliage of slippery elm is extremely rough, feeling like sandpaper, whereas white elm leaves are not as rough. As indicated in this old rural verse, the leaves also provide some guidance as to when to plant certain crops.

"When the elmen leaf is
as big as a mouse's ear, then
sow barley, never fear.
When elmen leaves are as big
as a penny, plant kidney beans
if you want to have any."

The fruit, known as samara, consist of a flat seed surrounded by a wing. This structure enables them to fly on the wind. White elm's corky bark has a spongy feel when pressed with your thumb, and once broken, it shows alternating layers of buff and dark brown colouration. The bark of slippery elm is a uniform dark, reddish-brown and retains this colour with weathering. The common name, red elm, and the botanical name *rubra* reflect the reddish characteristics of the bark.

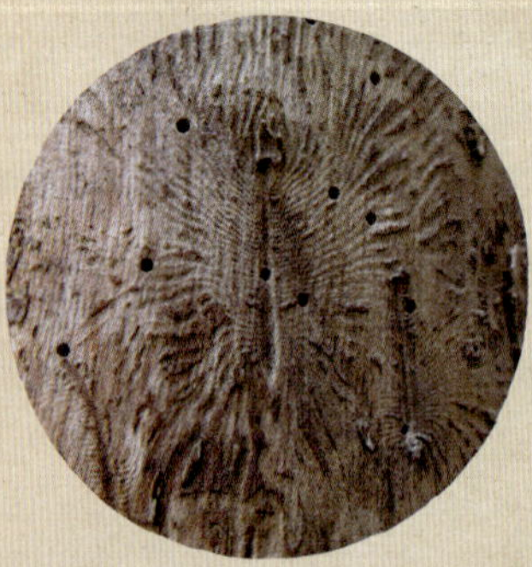

Egg chambers of elm bark beetle

Standing under an Elm

In North America it is felt that elms are full of good spirits; however, in parts of Europe, some consider that evil lurks in them. Elm trees are very stable and rarely blow down, even when growing out in open areas. However, the narrow crotches in their vase-shaped canopy create weak branching structure, making it treacherous to those below who linger too long. This is particularly true with wych elm (*Ulmus glabra*) and English elm (*Ulmus procera*), which have a reputation for dropping large branches not only in windstorms but also without warning on otherwise still days. Justifiably, such actions led to considerable distrust and those living in the English countryside became wary of the elm. A traditional saying was "the elm hateth man and waiteth." "I'll meet you under the elm" was another popular phrase in France, which was equivalent to the expression "when hell freezes over" and presumably indicated that it would be foolish to be caught loitering beneath an elm. On the other hand, traveling preachers would often speak beneath them to demonstrate their unwavering faith in God and to be sure their words were heard without being misunderstood.

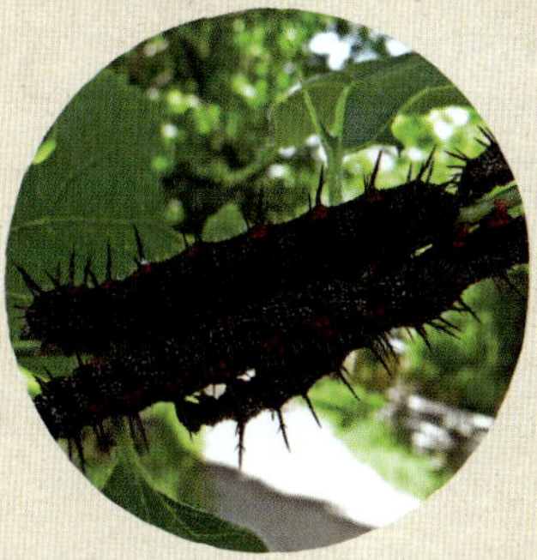

Spiny elm caterpillar

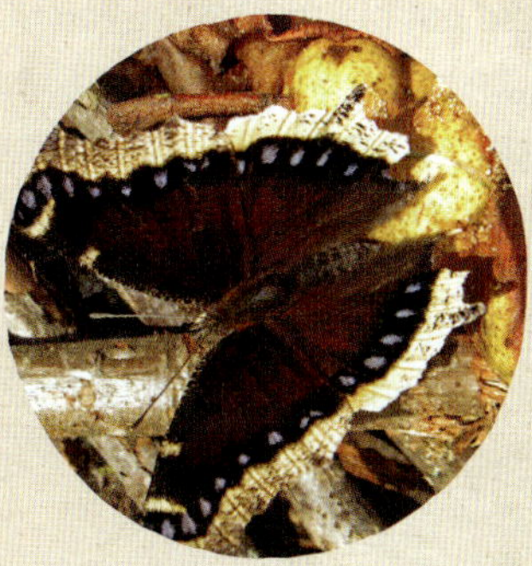

Mourning cloak butterfly

Dutch Elm Disease

Elms were a common feature in our woodlands, parks and along roads and fence lines until Dutch Elm Disease reached North America. It arrived in the United States from Europe in the 1930s, where it quickly spread. It came to Canada in 1944 in infected wooden crates, and within 15 years, six to seven million elms had died. Most of these "widow makers" met their demise in the '50s and '60s, and their dead skeletons that remained standing in the landscape were sad reminders of their legacy. Fortunately, elms appear to be making a comeback and at this time the tree is not in danger of extinction.

Wildlife Value

The expanding spring leaves attract and support the larvae of many *Lepidoptera* species, including the comma and question mark butterflies. Also common are masses of bristly black caterpillar with red dots known as the spiny elm caterpillar. These are the young of the mourning cloak butterfly, which overwinter as adults and are among our earliest spring butterflies.

The tree also attracts seed eaters, including song birds, rabbits and chipmunks, and the young leaves are consumed by porcupines and squirrels in spring. Slippery elm is particularly relished by twig browsers such as cottontails, white-tailed deer and porcupines, and the common name "moose elm" indicates that moose are fond of the young twigs and saplings. Orioles favour elms to build their bag nest at the end of the drooping branches. As well, woodpeckers excavate nesting cavities in dead elms and take advantage of the various insects that are found in the decaying wood.

Many morel species are associated with elms and are commonly found growing beneath the dead trees. After warm, humid weather, these fungi are harvested in spring and are considered a delicacy in the culinary world.

Culinary Uses

The inner bark of slippery elm has a mild, pleasant flavour with a faint licorice odour. It is very nutritious and easily digested, and when ground into a fine powder, it can be used as gruel to feed infants and patients whose systems need strengthening. It forms a wholesome food for those who are weak, debilitated, malnourished or convalescing after a long illness, helping to rebuild and nourish the body. It is high in healthful sugars, vitamins and minerals, including vitamin A and C, calcium, magnesium, phosphorus, potassium, selenium and zinc.

Elm bark was once ground into nutritious flour for making bread and remained part of the Laplanders' diet well into the nineteenth century. The Haudenosaunee (Iroquois) ate it in times of famine, and reports tell how George Washington's army survived the winter at Valley Forge by consuming the gruel. Twigs were chewed to help quench the thirst of travelers, and in the days before refrigeration, the bark was wrapped around meat to delay spoilage.

Medicinal Uses

Slippery elm bark is an old and beloved medicine among the North America Indigenous people and was quickly adopted by the early pioneers when they first arrived in this country. It became a fixture in home medicine cabinets, and by 1879 an ounce of powdered bark was worth ten cents in Canadian pharmacies. Considered the "official" elm in the American Pharmacopoeia, nothing compares to slippery elm's therapeutic qualities. It was once a common and versatile medicine that was close at hand until this great tree was decimated by Dutch Elm Disease. It continues to play an important role in herbal medicine, but ethical harvesting techniques should be followed.

It is slippery elm's excellent demulcent and emollient benefits that make this a valuable herbal remedy. Its principal asset is the abundant slimy mucilage found within the inner bark, and by coating and moistening all parts it comes in direct contact with, it acts to soothe and protect tissues and exposed surfaces. As with many herbs containing mucilage, it has a predictable influence on the mucosa of the digestive, respiratory and urinary systems, promoting lubrication, cleansing, strengthening and healing. It doesn't have a direct toning effect, but instead helps reduce inflammation and penetrates the tissues and cells to bring out toxins. Used both externally and internally, its soothing qualities make it extremely valuable for healing wounds, burns, skin inflammation, coughs, sore throats and digestive problems, including peptic ulcers. Slippery elm is also one of the four ingredients in the famous Essiac formula, promoted by Canadian nurse Rene Caisse as an herbal treatment for cancer.

The pleasant-tasting inner bark swells in water to become gelatinous or slippery. It is mild but very effective, and a small spoonful constitutes a medicinal dose. The bark is collected in early spring when the sap begins to flow and should be gathered with environmental ethics in mind. This classic remedy is available commercially as lozenge, tea or in powdered form to be used either internally or as a poultice. Adulteration is common. The powder should be a light, tawny colour, not dark or reddish. After stirring it into cold water to make a paste, add hot water and let it sit, then add it to drinks, oatmeal, yogurt or smoothies. Be aware that the mucilage may interfere with absorption of other medication.

Digestion

Like marshmallow root, the mucilaginous properties in slippery elm bark help to temporarily coat and sooth the stomach and intestinal lining, offering relief from numerous digestive complaints. Its demulcent qualities help ease irritation of the mucous membrane and promote the healing of inflamed and damaged tissues. The mucilage is very resistant to digestive juices; therefore, the demulcent action continues down the lining of the digestive tract, benefiting the entire system as it passes through. This explains its use for quickly easing gastritis, ulcerations and colitis. It also helps neutralize excess stomach acid to relieve heartburn and other irritations resulting from hyperacidity.

Gentle enough for children, it is employed for bowel issues and has

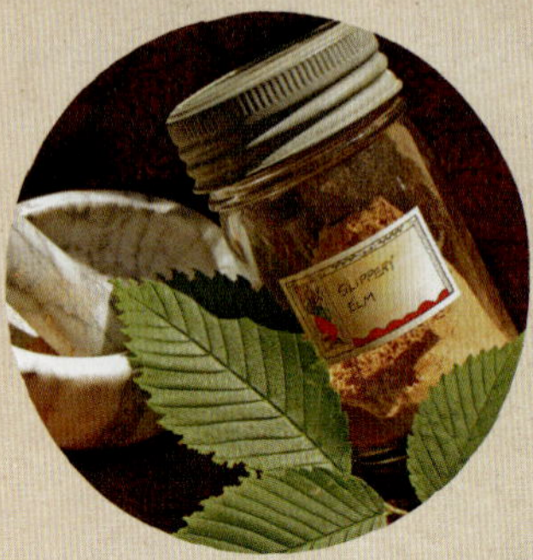

Powdered bark of slippery elm

proven useful as both a laxative and a treatment for diarrhea. In 1834 Dr. John Eberle wrote that it exerts a specific action in dysentery and chronic diarrhea and its effects are "so immediate that it appears like a charm." However, he does go on to say that its healing virtues may not be explained by its demulcent action alone, for other demulcents do not produce the same healing results. It continues to be used with great results for severe dysentery with cramping pain and to reduce intestinal inflammation. Additionally, elm helps keep the digestive tract lubricated and moist to ensure everything continues to move smoothly. By soothing the intestinal lining and softening hard stools, it eases constipation and restores healthy bowel movements. These same principles also make it useful for treating hemorrhoids, where it is employed both internally and externally.

Because it absorbs toxins in the digestive tract, it is valued in the management of food poisoning. Furthermore, the sugars in the inner bark stimulate and enhance the growth and reproduction of beneficial bacteria that live in the large intestines, thus encouraging healthy digestion.

Respiratory System

As valuable throat and lung medicine, slippery elm is employed for all types of respiratory conditions, and at one time elm lozenges were a fixture in home medicine cabinets. Its demulcent properties make it particularly useful for easing dry, irritating coughs and soothing sore throats. It greatly benefits bronchitis, pneumonia, tuberculosis and other lung afflictions, and is often utilized in colds and asthma because it deepens respiration and rids mucus.

Wound Remedy

In *Materia Medica America*, written in 1797, slippery elm was known as "salve bark," and for good reason. Its primary assets are its emollient actions, where the mucilage coats surfaces, thereby producing soothing and protective qualities. This makes it an important wound remedy, helping to ease pain, irritation and itching, and to bind torn and damaged tissues. It also reduces swelling and assists in drawing out pus.

Historically, slippery elm was used for all types of tumors, rashes and inflamed surfaces with great results, and many herbalists still claim its healing abilities make it the best possible poultice for dressing fresh wounds, burns, boils, abscesses and ulcers. The Native Americans regularly wrapped the bark around injuries of flesh and bone, and in 1830 Rafinesque noted that during the American Revolution (1765 to 1783), slippery elm poultices were the chief means of treating gunshot wounds to help extract the balls. By the mid-1800s, it was such an important remedy of the European settlers that it could be found in almost any drug store. The coarsely ground bark, which was mixed with water to make a paste, was placed on wounds, and when dried formed an herbal bandage.

Bones and Joints

Because slippery elm is particularly effective at resolving dryness of tissues, it has an important influence on the synovial membranes in joints that have dried out, making it useful for numerous bone and joint ailments. A poultice works nicely on carpal tunnel syndrome when applied daily for one hour for a week. Furthermore, it was employed for fractured limbs, as it "healeth broken bones very speedily if they be fomented or bathed there in."

The First Nations peoples put the powder into a hollow tooth to stop the ache and greatly deter deterioration. This remedy is still useful for reducing cavities and should be utilized as soon as there is any sign of decay.

Birthing

Slippery elm was well known to Indigenous women for assisting childbirth and to moisten and lubricate the passage during labour. Samuel Henry (1814) and Rafinesque (1828) both recommended it for pregnant women during the last two months of their pregnancy to facilitate the birth and instigate a speedy and easy delivery.

Use of the Wood

An old forester once told me that elms are "the most useless piece of vegetation in our forest." It is inadequate as firewood because it is challenging to split and full of water; it is unsuitable as building material since it warps and twists readily; it is unfit for posts due to the fact that it rots quickly, and on top of this, it gives off an unpleasant odor. However, elm wood does have some redeeming qualities.

Kipling wrote, "Ailim be the lady's tree, burn it not or cursed ye'll be." To firewood operators, elm wood can indeed be frustrating. Its twisted, interlocking grain is laid down in a cross-hatch pattern, making it difficult, if not impossible, to split. However, this characteristic gives the wood strength, and if allowed to cure, it burns with great heat. As well, elm has the distinct ability to hold nails without spitting them back out, and when sawn across the twisted grain, an attractive pattern known as "partridge breast" is revealed.

Although the wood distorts easily, it is tough, durable, very flexible and resistant to splitting. This made it useful for wagons, heavy sleighs, cutters and truck floors, and farmers often had both elm and ash on hand to put to use when a strong, hard wood was needed for small articles, such as axe helves, tool handles, wheel hubs, spokes, harrows and yokes for oxen. Like ash, elm is also highly resistant to shock. This renders it beneficial for articles that are required to withstand impact, such as sporting equipment and chopping blocks, and it was the traditional pedestal for blacksmith anvils.

One of the earliest uses of elm's flexible wood was in bow making, and it was considered the next best material, after yew. In fact, some of the oldest artifacts in Europe, dating around 2800 BC, are Danish flat bows made of elm wood. Gerald of Wales, a thirteenth-century Anglo-Norman nobleman who wrote extensively on Welsh customs, noted that the archers of South Wales made their long bows with wych elm (wych being an ancient word referring to its pliability), while English bowmen favoured yew (*Taxus baccata*). The yews used were often harvested from churchyards. Because yews are poisonous to animals, they were planted behind the walls surrounding places of worship so that animals could graze freely outside the stone barriers. They were not only used to fashion bows; it was also believed that walking around a yew seven times would grant a wish. Paths were worn around the branches of old yews from people regularly performing these rituals.

Another redeeming quality of elm wood is that it is very resistant in wet situations when not exposed to alternating wet and dry conditions. In this fluctuating environment the wood is classified as "non-durable" and rots rapidly, making the wood unsuitable for items like fence posts or exterior work. Nonetheless, it is quite water resistant and can survive for centuries underground and in water when not exposed to air. This renders it an excellent choice for boat hulls and keels, wharves, bridge foundations, pilings and canal lock gates. In the early 1600s, London, England's urban water system was constructed with elm pipes before the introduction of metal. Most of this underground plumbing, when unearthed in the 1930s, was still sound, having withstood 300 years below ground. The wood was also traditionally used for making coffins and likely played this role due to its durability beneath the soil.

White elm's unpleasant odor is similar to that of urine, and displeased colonists called it "piss elm." However, this refers to the green wood; when dried it is relatively odourless and well suited for crates and barrels to hold fruit and vegetables.

Useful Bark

In the past, the North American Indigenous people utilized the corky, buoyant bark of elm more than its wood. Noted in many diaries of European travelers during the fifteenth and sixteenth centuries, one of its main roles was in the construction of bark canoes. While the Ojibway (Anishinaabe) made their canoes from birch bark, the Iroquois (Haudenosaunee) were forced to use elm, since birch did not grow abundantly in their region. In spring, when the sap was running, the bark was easily stripped from the tree in a large single sheet. It was turned inside out, so that the smooth inner surface became the exterior of the canoe, and was then stretched around a frame of bent ash ribs to shape the vessel.

These strong, sturdy boats did not capsize easily and were well suited for heavy loads of meats and skins. However, compared to the sleek, state-of-the-art birch back canoes of the Anishinaabe, elm bark canoes were significantly heavier and slower, and their neighbours literally left them sitting in the water.

The Indigenous peoples covered their wigwams and shingled their long houses and meeting houses with elm bark. The United Empire Loyalists who settled around Kingston, Ontario, in the late 1700s also made their cabin roofs with elm bark. The bark was laid in overlapping layers to form a covering that kept out wind and weather.

Bark containers of various shapes and sizes were made by the Indigenous women to hold water and gather maple sap in spring. These same vessels, known as *makuks*, were later used to store maple sugar. Kettles for stewing meat were also constructed from elm bark. The containers, holding both meat and water, were suspended over the fire and the meat would be nicely cooked before the kettle burnt through.

Depicted in Paintings

Elm's fanning branches have a distinctive shape that artists love to draw, and it was prominently featured in many famous English and American paintings. English painter John Constable was particularly noted for his portrayals of elms, and the elm is commemorated in the art of AJ Casson and Quebec painter Marc-Aurele Fortin. There are many renowned portraits of celebrated men standing beneath an elm, and Donald Culross once wrote, "If you want to be recalled for something that you do, you will be well advised to do it under an elm."

Treaty Elms

Negotiations during council and community meetings were held under the sweeping boughs of elms, and treaties were signed beneath them. Appropriately, trees under which these agreements were endorsed were called "Treaty Elms" and historic plaques indicate where they once stood. Most notably, William Penn's legendary treaty between the European settlers and the Delaware natives to colonize Pennsylvania was signed beneath an ancient elm in 1682. This historical event was commemorated by Benjamin West in his famous painting *Penn Treaty with the Indians*. There is no firm evidence of this treaty's existence, nor is it known what the terms were. It is rumoured that Penn's "Treaty Elm" blew down in 1810 on the banks of the Delaware River. Another noted elm was the tree under which George Washington took command of the continental army in 1775.

Folklore

The *Iliad*, an epic poem by the ancient Greek poet Homer (written in eighth century BC) that recounted some of the significant events of the Trojan War, was believed to contain the first literary reference of elms being planted at the tombs of soldiers to honor those who tragically died at war. The elm tree was also credited with saving the great warrior Achilles from drowning as he grasped a branch of a great elm.

Among the Anglo-Saxons, elms were once called "elven wood" because they were associated with the spirit world and had a particularly affinity to wood elves. These mythological beings were said to guard the dead, burial mounds, and the passage to the underworld. They posed as a connection between the living and the dead and would appear under an elm after a long night of music and festivities. It was thought that to strengthen your relationship with wood elves, one should bond with an elm by bringing it gifts and spending time with it.

If a small piece of the bark was hung around a child's neck, it helped them learn a language and ensured persuasive speaking skills later in life—perhaps bringing us back to judges and courts.

Carrying slippery elm was said to make the bearer impervious to slander and was used to stop malicious gossip and the spreading of lies. By throwing some into a fire, any harmful things said about you would cease. It protected you from jealous co-workers, covetous neighbours and hidden enemies posing as friends. It was rumoured that placing a small pinch of the powder in the corners of rooms protected the home and rid the premises of evil.

Lessons of Elm

Elm has wonderful spiritual qualities that offer defense and protection, especially when it comes to family and those you love. Like an umbrella, she shields you when life brings rain and provides fortification during times of adversity. She is steadfast and loyal, bringing justice into your life and helping you endure when faced with daunting obstacles. She is the counsel that listens without judgment.

Life's difficulties can create the illusion that we are isolated and alone, leaving us feeling powerless and trapped. Elm's gentle spirit encourages us to rethink a situation from a different perspective and inspires us to look at it honestly, so that we can see the greater picture. She helps you speak from the heart and express yourself without being misunderstood, and she ensures others are conveying the truth and being honest with you.

Hawthorn

Crataegus sp.

May, May Tree, May Bush, May Haw, May Blossom, Mayflower, Haw, Hedge Thorn, Hag Thorn, Whitethorn, Quick Thorn, Quickset, Pixie Pears, Cuckoo's Beads, Thorn Apples, Apple Haw, Holy Thorn, Christ's Crown, Bread and Cheese and Ladies' Meat

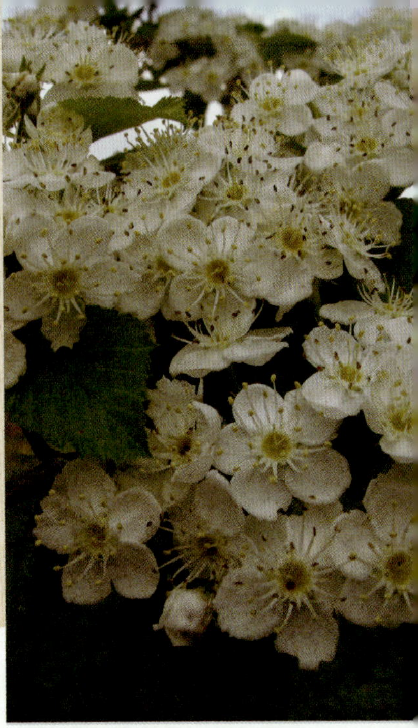

In North America, most have little appreciation or fondness for hawthorns, considering them an insignificant feature in our environment. Indeed, more often than not, landowners inquire about their eradication rather than their preservation. However, in other parts of the world, these sacred trees are revered and respected, beloved by fairies and all those who believe in love and magic. This delightful tree brings lovers, playmates, joy and fun into our lives.

Under the Protection of Fairies

In Great Britain and Ireland, hawthorns are still cherished as trees of enchantment, and it is believed that where they reside, friendly spirits gather. Isolated hawthorns, called "lone bushes," are common in fields and on burial mounds and are considered to be the most likely tree inhabited by fairies. Being under the protection of the wee folk, they are fiercely defended and are never cut or harmed in any way without the fear of incurring the wrath of their guardians. Indeed, in Ireland, farmers still plough around them and roads continue to be rerouted to ensure their safety. If it is deemed absolutely necessary to remove a hawthorn, it is customary to give it three days warning to allow the tree spirits to move elsewhere.

Meeting Hawthorn

Hawthorns are able to survive poor soils and high winds, providing a protective presence in barren landscapes. Being shade-intolerant, this pioneer species needs full sun to develop and tends to grow alone or in even-aged thickets in old fields, open woods and hedge rows. This native tree is not invasive, but neither does it allow itself to become invaded, as it finds a way to adapt and hold its ground. Because it is able to compete with thick sod, it is one of the first trees to start a forest ecosystem and an important nurse tree in our environment. As it slowly shades out competitive grasses and forbs, it leads the way for other tree seedlings to follow, allowing them to take their place in the landscape. Once these species become established, the hawthorn is soon shaded out and replaced.

Due to the fact they frequently hybridize, many species and sub-species exist in Canada. Nonetheless, as a group, these small, elegant trees in the rose family, whose trunks and branches become twisted with age, are easily distinguished by their long, spear-like thorns and the bright-red or yellow berries. Throughout the year, they make a nice show in garden settings, from their glorious spring flowers and colourful fall fruit, to the light gray skeleton of bare branches in winter.

Hawthorn's apple-like blossoms are white with yellow centers, providing a spectacular spring display. The trees are most prominent while in bloom and reveal their glory by forming beautiful white swaths across the rural landscape. The scent of the blossoms varies, with some species having very little fragrance while others suggest the odour of decomposing matter or decaying fish. Due to the smell, the flowers attract carrion flies and beetles, which in turn assist in pollination. During Medieval Europe, it was considered unlucky to bring hawthorn flowers into the house, as this could result in the death or illness of a family member. For many villagers, the unpleasant aroma indicated that the flowers still bore the smell of the Great Plague of London. Chemists have now discovered that a chemical in hawthorn blossoms is also one of the first chemicals formed in decaying

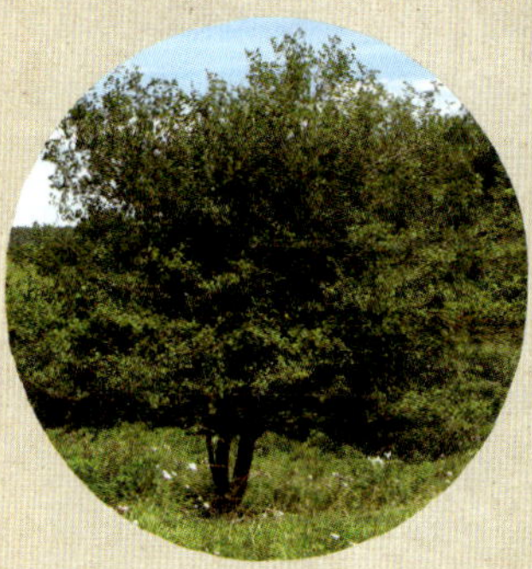

Isolated hawthorns are fiercely protected by the fairies

animal tissue, so it is not surprising that they were not welcome in homes.

On the other hand, hawthorn blossoms were also associated with the Blessed Virgin Mary, and shrines devoted to her were decorated with "May" blossoms. The Druids also honoured hawthorn, believing the white flowers denoted the maiden aspect of the triple goddess, while the glowing red fruit of fall represented the mother and the bare branches of winter the crone.

The Arrival of Spring

Another name for hawthorn is the "May Tree," and according to the Celts, it was the blooming of this tree that announced the true arrival of spring. The beautiful white blossoms marked the end of the dark winter, giving cause to celebrate nature's renewal of life. The English saying "cast ne'er a clout 'til May is out" meant that one should not put away their winter clothing until the hawthorn was in bloom, not at the end of May as this adage first seems to imply.

Meaning of its Name

The term haw and hag are old English words for hedge; thus, the very name hawthorn or hag thorn translates into hedge thorn. Because of their long, sharp spines, these trees were valued for fast growing, impenetrable hedges or live barriers to divide fields and contain livestock. It was, and still is, the most common species in hedgerows throughout the countryside of the British Isles. Maybe because of this, thorn is the most frequently used tree in English place names, with examples being Thorndale, Thornbury and Thornhill.

Because of the red fruit, in some areas it is known as pixie pears, cuckoo's beads or thorn apples, and the light-coloured bark gave it the name whitethorn. Holy thorn or Christ's crown refers to the belief that the branches formed Christ's crown of thorns at his crucifixion, and as a result hawthorn became both feared and regarded as sacred. As well, the Mayflower, the boat in which the first Pilgrims came to North America, was thought to be named after the English hawthorn (*Crataegus monogyna*).

Wildlife Value

Mice, deer and bears are fond of the fruit. As well, a number of bird species occasionally eat the haws and like cherries, the fermented fruit can sometimes make our feathered friends intoxicated during warm, wet falls. The flowers attract carrion flies and beetles and the pollen and nectar are much sought-after by honeybees. When grown in gardens and around

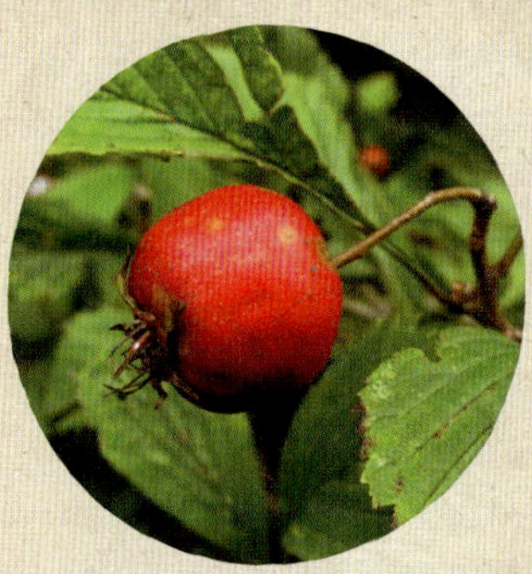

The fruit is made into jelly, syrup and cold drinks

fields, hawthorns draw in beneficial insects and song birds, thus reducing the need for pesticides.

It is the long, pointed thorns, however, that provide the most benefit to wildlife. This small tree provides excellent protection and cover to conceal the nests of song birds and these homes become obvious in winter when they are revealed in the bare branches.

Watch for the loggerhead shrike (a species at risk in Ontario) when strolling through hawthorn thickets. Their diet consists mostly of large insects, frogs, small birds, voles and mice, but their hunting and feeding methods are unique. Unlike hawks, these birds have no grasping talons, so they impale their prey on thorns or wedge it in tree crotches to make consumption easier. The males may also lodge their food on thorns or barbed wire fences to display their competence at hunting, as a territorial display or to store excess food during times of plenty. If there is a variety of skewered critters baking in the sun, it is an indication that loggerhead shrikes are present. A decline in their population is believed to be from habitat destruction and a lack of old fields with hawthorns. Grey squirrels have also been seen impaling mushrooms and apples on the thorns, storing and drying them for future use.

Culinary Uses

The small apple-like fruit, known as haws, are high in vitamin C and antioxidants. The seeds have been found during archaeological digs, suggesting that for many centuries the fruit was used as food. This tradition continues, and today locals from Manitoulin Island, Ontario, hold haw festivals every fall and fondly call themselves haw-eaters. The fruit varies widely in taste and texture, with some species being sweetish-sour and juicy, others dry and bland. Most make a nice apple-like jelly or syrup when cooked with sugar and they contain plenty of their own pectin. Hawthorn wine is quite popular, and an excellent liqueur with an exquisite taste can be made from the berries or flowers when infused in brandy. The steeped fruit also make a nice tea or cold drink.

North American Indigenous peoples cooked, then dried the fruit on birch bark and formed them into cakes to be used throughout the winter in soups or as an addition to pemmican. Over in Europe, a type of bread was made from the ground, dried fruit; thus, the haws were sometimes known as "flour berries." The young leaves were frequently nibbled by children, who nicknamed them "bread and cheese," and in times of hardship they were eaten by European peasants to fill their empty bellies.

Medicinal Uses

Hawthorn has been embraced as one of the best remedies for the heart and blood vessels. Its beneficial actions were mentioned by Greek physician Dioscorides in the first century but it didn't gain popularity in Europe to treat cardiovascular disorders until the 1800s. During the Victorian time period, hawthorn was utilized by Doctor Green of Clare County, Ireland, to successfully treat heart disease; however, he never revealed the secret of his remedy. Upon his death in 1894, his daughter disclosed that the medicine he had been using was indeed hawthorn berries. Doctor J.C. Jennings of Chicago took his findings and wrote an article for the New York Medical Journal in 1896, promoting its use for a variety of heart problems. From here it became well known, benefiting almost every aspect of cardiovascular health.

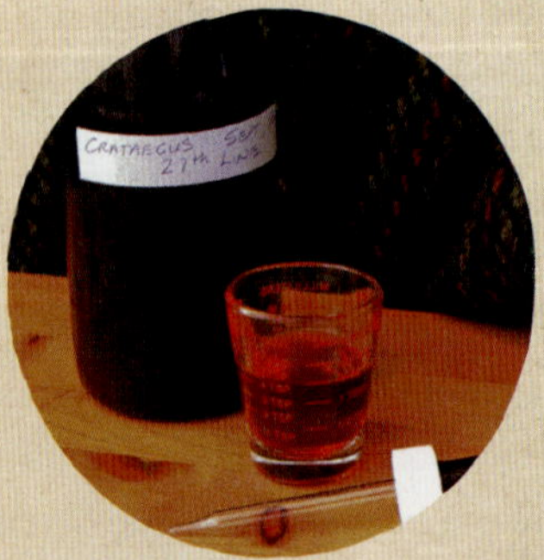

Hawthorn tincture

The deep, blood-red colour of the fruit is often taken as an indication of its healing properties. However, it is not only the berries, but also the flowers and new leaves that provide us with one of the best tonics for the circulatory system. Modern research has verified its use, proving useful in increasing the efficiency of the heart muscle, opening coronary and peripheral circulation, regulating blood pressure, lowering unhealthy cholesterol levels and combating the effects of arteriosclerosis and congestive heart failure.

It works slowly and should be taken over an extended period to produce noticeable results. It is recommended for aging men, and it is rumored that if a woman truly loves her husband, she will start giving him hawthorn when he turns 40 to keep his heart healthy and strong. A tea, cordial or jelly is an enjoyable way to take this medicine.

Medicine for the Heart

A number of properties provide hawthorn its medicinal qualities. Its astringent action has a toning effect on the blood vessels, improving circulation and removing congestion associated with heat. Rich in flavonoids, it helps dilate the blood vessels and increase their flexibility, thereby releasing cardiovascular constriction so that blood and oxygen flow more freely through the entire system. Furthermore, its antispasmodic properties and antioxidants offer a profound healing effect by relaxing and nourishing the heart muscle. Together these virtues protect and strengthen a weakened heart, allowing it to beat more forcefully and efficiently, and increasing the amount of blood pumped with each contraction. This in turn helps regulate the blood pressure, resulting in less strain on the heart. Improved circulation can also help lift confusion and forgetfulness that comes with inadequate blood supply to the brain.

Hawthorn has an amazing ability to normalize the heart by stimulating or depressing its activity depending upon its need. It moves the heart to normal function in a gentle and supportive way, by either calming a rapid heartbeat or regulating a slow, weak one. It can be included in a personal regime to forestall future heart and circulation problems or to enhance the heart during exercise. It is also a wonderful herb to improve athletic performance by toning and opening the capillary bed.

As a remarkable herb for both preventing and treating heart disease, hawthorn brings vitality and support to the heart muscle weakened or degenerated by age and is restorative after a heart attack. It helps a senile heart that has forgotten how to function properly and makes it more efficient by increasing cardiac performance. Some of hawthorn's most impressive and best research benefits are to prevent, treat and potentially reverse the early symptoms of congestive heart failure, such as chronic fatigue, shortness of breath and fluid congestion around the heart, as well as alleviate chest pains and discomfort due to mild, stable forms of angina. It can also be used to help reduce nervous palpitations and anxiety that sometimes accompany heart conditions.

Furthermore, the extended use of

hawthorn has been reputed to have a normalizing effect on cholesterol by both lowering unhealthy amounts from the blood stream and maintaining healthy levels. Its antioxidants have been shown to effectively dissolve and inhibit the buildup of plaque on injured blood vessels, thus reducing the risk of arteriosclerosis, or hardening of the arteries. This condition is characterized by deposits developing in the arteries, causing loss of elasticity and thickening of the walls. When plaque becomes loose in the blood stream it can rapidly lead to a blockage, resulting in a heart attack or stroke.

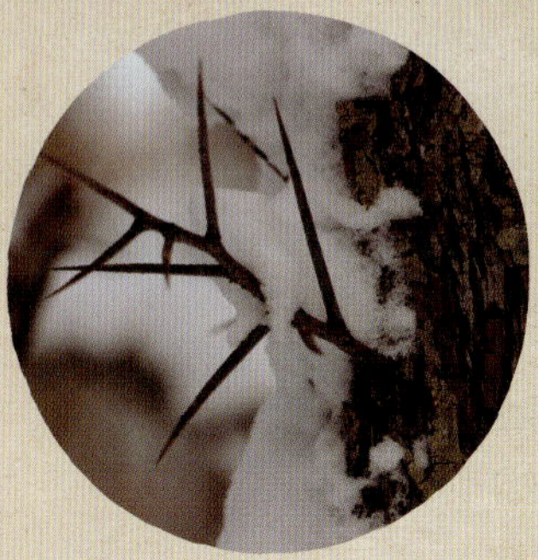

The sharp spines of hawthorn

Other Medicinal Uses

In Europe, hawthorn was sometimes called "ladies' meat," as it was once customary to cook the berries with meat to make it more digestible. Hawthorn works to promote a sluggish digestion by strengthening the blood vessels in the digestive tract and increasing gastric enzymes. Its high vitamin C content also led to its use in treating scurvy, a disease caused from a deficiency of this vitamin. Moreover, it may relieve kidney and bladder problems by increasing urination and dissolving deposits.

Hawthorn also has a calming effect on the emotions, proving useful for reducing anxiety, menopausal mood swings, restlessness, nervous tension and insomnia. By relaxing the nervous system and heart, it can be used in cases of attention deficit and overactive children, helping them focus and settle down.

If one is scratched or pricked by the thorn, it will cause an infection or inflammation. An Indigenous medicine woman once said, "There is something in the thorn that causes the skin not to heal when it is pricked, but if you pick that thorn and prick a boil, it will empty out and heal up."

Tree for Beauty

At one time, young women would rise at dawn on the first of May to bathe their faces in the dew of the hawthorn blossoms, giving them eternal beauty. This is affirmed in this little verse:

The fair maid who, the first of May
Goes to the fields at break of day

And washes in dew from
the hawthorn tree
Will ever after handsome be

Hawthorn's Wood of Love

The botanical name *Crataegus,* comes from the Greek word *kratos,* meaning strength, which describes the remarkable toughness of the wood. Making one of the hottest fires, it is excellent for fuel, especially in cook stoves. On the morn of May 1, the first smoke to go up the chimney should be that of hawthorn or rowan, to ensure no harm comes to the family.

The hard wood has little commercial value due to the tree's small size; however, it has a fine, close grain that takes on a beautiful polish and was traditionally used for making small articles such as walking sticks, knife handles, small jewelry boxes, hair ornaments, combs and other talismans. Being a symbol of the heart, these gifts of hawthorn wood were considered "trinkets of love" and given as a token of friendship and endearment.

Other Uses

At one time the thorns were used as fishing hooks, awls and needles for sewing, and carrying a hawthorn spine on fishing trips was thought to ensure a good catch. In autumn, young children would search out the haws and, after sucking the thick skin from the hard seeds, they would use the stones in their blowguns and pop-guns.

Sacred Groves

Being one of their favourite trees, witches were often seen dancing beneath their branches, and most gardens belonging to old hedge herbalists contained at least one hawthorn. In the British Isles, this sacred tree was considered to have powerful magical influences, and pagans worshiped and performed rituals in groves of hawthorns. Later, Christian churches were built on these locations, and it is alleged that Westminster Abbey stands where a sacred grove of thorn trees once grew.

Protecting Springs and Wells

The connection of wells and hawthorns was an important one. In English villages, as late as the early 1900s, it was customary to decorate wells from which the community drew their water starting on Ascension Day (40 days after Easter) until the end of August. This came from an ancient pagan practice that originated as a ritual of thanksgiving and remembrance for the gift of clean, clear water. Believing that good spirits would only abide in wells if they were remembered and respectfully addressed, people brought offerings of flowers, green branches and other gifts, and festivals and dances were carried out. Hawthorns were thought to guard the place where water came from the earth, keeping it pure. Therefore, it was also common practice to plant them near their water sources, and many thorns continue to flourish where old wells and springs were located. Ribbons or wish rags are still tied to these sacred thorns to bring luck, love and happiness.

A Symbol of Fertility and Love

Bearing white spring flowers and red berries in fall, hawthorn became a symbol of fertility and love. To the Greeks and Romans, it represented happiness and was particularly linked to sweet hope, marriages and fruitfulness. It found its place in spring weddings to bring abundance to the new couple, and the flowering branches were carried in marriage processions. The Celts associated it with courtship and often presented the flowers to their "friend of the heart."

Furthermore, on the morning of Samhain (Halloween), men went to their fields, armed with plenty of beer and cider, to kindle small fires of hawthorn to bless and enhance the fertility of the wheat fields for the upcoming growing season. It is said the custom was so widely observed that the whole countryside "twinkled like stars" in the darkness of the early morning.

Tree of Protection

Perhaps due to their sharp spines, hawthorns were planted near homes and barns to provide protection. The branches, which were sprinkled with holy water, were put into the ground around field edges to prevent the fairies from taking the crops and were hung over doorways in hopes of keeping away negative energy and ensuring no ghosts could enter.

Although ash and oak were thought to attract lightning, sitting under the hawthorn was rumoured to protect you from its wrath, as noted in this verse:

Beware the oak, it draws the stroke
Avoid the ash, it courts the flash
Creep under the thorn, it
will save you from harm

For generations, many have come to her for shelter, and when planted in gardens hawthorns were believed to be powerful protectors from damaging storms and lightning strikes. To add further insurance, its wood was sometimes incorporated into buildings during construction.

Lessons of the Hawthorn

Hawthorn's energy has the ability to center us and let us stand our ground when we feel that we are being pulled in every direction. This allows us to stay in touch with the present and all the opportunities it has to offer.

Hawthorn has long represented the heart, and in the *Language of Flowers* it signifies hope. It is reputed for its ability to heal the heart on every level, not only physically but also by influencing its emotional and spiritual aspects. It is thought to cheer the soul and promote happiness, making it a wonderful remedy for mending "broken hearts." By calming the nerves and lifting the mood, it helps resolve deep feelings of sorrow and grief and is specific for those who have a difficult time expressing their feelings or releasing their emotions. It defends the spirit and reminds the heart who you are, allowing us to let go of the past and bring forgiveness and healing. Keeping the heart light, free and open to love is hawthorn's gift.

Hemlock

Tsuga canadensis

Eastern Hemlock, Canada Hemlock, Hemlock Spruce and Sore-Healing Woman

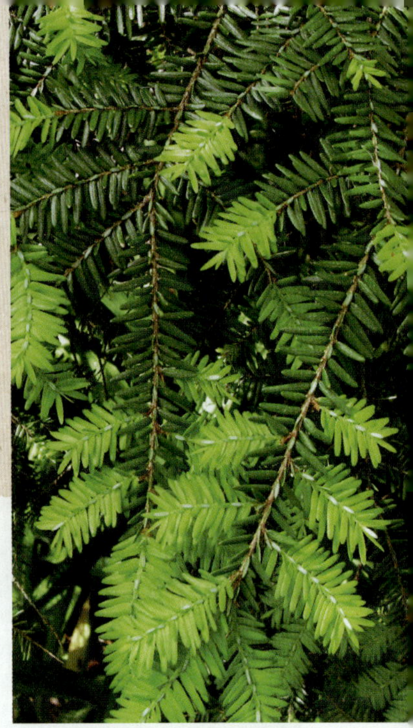

On hot, humid days I head to the hemlocks, for there is no cooler sanctuary from the summer heat. On cold wintery days, I also seek out a hemlock, to sit under her soft branches, sheltered and protected from wind and snow. The dense, feathery needles, which give this tree its graceful form, provide fortification to those beneath. In 1698, Father Louis Hennepin, stationed on Lake Ontario, claimed hemlocks are "the prettiest trees in the world." Indeed, this native evergreen is one of the most elegant; from her soft, lacy boughs that gently droop, to her small but abundant cones that adorn her branches like jewels. Its evergreen features denote the promise of spring, supporting us through the winter months.

Meeting Hemlock

This very ancient tree is in the pine family (*Pinaceae*) and native to northeastern North America. It once grew in northern Europe; however, the only traces of hemlock left in this prehistoric location are deeply buried in fossil form. Slow growing and long lived, the eastern hemlock can attain a substantial size and is often found in old growth forests. It starts its life as an understory tree, growing in the shade of others, but eventually becomes one of the tallest in the woods, reaching heights of 30 to 35 meters (100 to 115 feet) and diameters of 1.5 meters (5 feet). Often dominating the landscape, it towers over others and specimens were once used as landmarks by travelers. Being a tree that prefers cool, moist woodlands, they frequently grow on north facing slopes, particularly in ravines and valleys bordering rivers, streams and lakes. In these habitats,

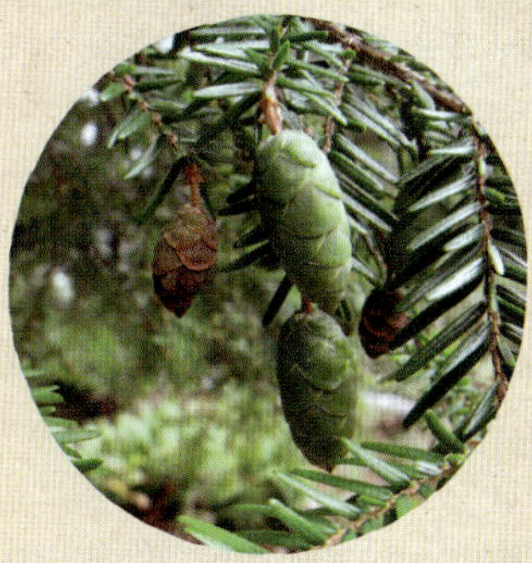

Cones that adorn her branches like jewels

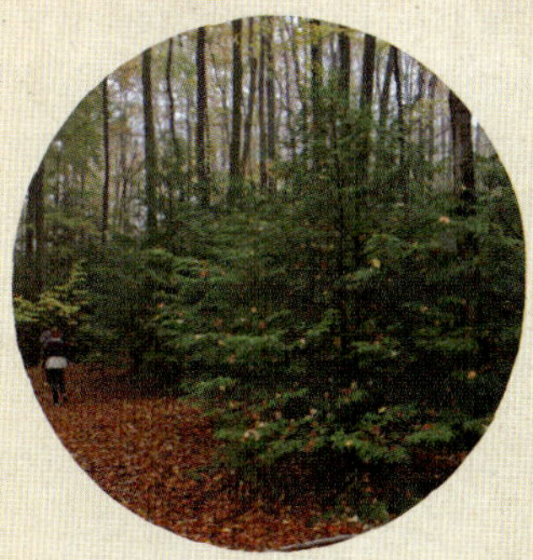

Hemlocks are found scattered among deciduous trees

their strong roots help prevent soil erosion, thus improving water quality and maintaining healthy spawning beds. Despite their longevity, hemlocks have low tolerance for pollution and road salt, and their shallow, sensitive roots are easily damaged by ground fires, droughts, compaction and disturbance from human intrusion. It favours sheltered locations away from drying winds and the heat of the sun.

Shade Tolerance

Being very shade tolerant, the young hemlock trees are able to grow very slowly in low light for many decades until a sunny opening is created. It is a tree of patience, biding its time under its larger neighbours, and once a gap is formed it quickly reaches into the canopy. This majestic tree can live 400 to 500 years if it does not succumb to disease, insects or pollution, although much older specimens exist, with some approaching 1000 years. Due to her longevity, hemlocks hold our history and stories of the past. "A monument of bygone days, I've kept the place where now I grow"—a segment of poem from the book *The Hemlock Tree and Its Legends* (1959) by Robert Bradbury—speaks of these attributes.

However, hemlock's thick, overlapping foliage also casts some of the densest shade of any tree. It creates its own dark, acidic microenvironment, allowing little to grow beneath. Indeed, their shade is so dark their own seedlings have difficulties getting a start. For this reason, hemlocks rarely grow in pure stands, but instead, are found scattered among hardwoods such as sugar maples, yellow birch and beech, where light can filter through. Thus, trees of all sizes and ages can be found dotted around the trunks of mature deciduous trees.

In the Garden

Bradbury also wrote in *The Hemlock Tree and Its Legend* that, "In every branch I have a tongue; I have a voice in every breeze." Perhaps it is the whispering sounds, or the graceful branches accentuated with bobbing cones as they dance in the wind, that leads to the admiration for hemlock among gardeners. It is valued in the landscape trade as an attractive evergreen that tolerates shady conditions. Few trees are more elegant, and its dark, rich, green foliage remains unchanged through the year, making it ideal in winter landscapes.

Association with Fungi and Mycorrhiza

As a species, hemlock grows in a singular fashion, well-spaced from fellow trees. However, when it comes to other species, they are very gregarious, often living and thriving in close proximity with deciduous trees. Their shallow roots seem not to compete with their deciduous companions, which often put down roots deeper in the rooting zone. Furthermore, hemlocks are associated with a great diversity of fungal and mycelium species which are capable of mineral solubility. The fungal threads grow into the soft root hairs, thereby increasing the root surface so that considerably more water and nutrients can be absorbed by the tree. The two organisms work together to form a partnership. The fungus roams the forest floor, picking up moisture and nutrients, such as nitrogen and phosphorus, which it then provides to the tree. In return, the hemlock provides sugar to the fungus for its services. Recent studies have also shown that minerals are also being exchanged between the hemlocks and their neighbours, thus granting some nutrients to their deciduous counterpart.

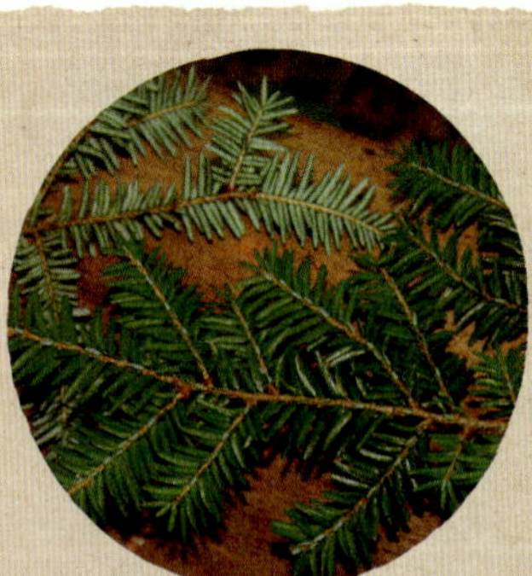

Needles make a pleasant tea

Hemlock also plays host to a number of mushrooms found in northern temperate forests. Even in death, this tree continues to heal, for the well-known rishi mushroom, *Ganaderma tsugae*, can be found growing on dead or dying hemlock trunks. The bright, red, kidney-shaped cap and varnished appearance makes this showy polypore quite distinct. *Ganaderma* contains polysaccharides known to have medicinal properties that have long been recognized in Chinese medicine. Today, it is suggested that it boosts immunity and benefits as an alternative adjunct to conventional cancer treatments.

Wildlife Value

Because of their flexible branches, hemlocks endure snow well, bending and bowing without breaking. They allow little snow to fall beneath them, providing protection to a variety of wildlife. White tailed deer often "yard up" in hemlock stands during heavy snow falls, where they are sheltered from the elements and can enjoy a meal on the foliage. Many birds nest in their branches, and black-capped chickadees, juncos, crossbills and pine siskins feed on their oil-rich seeds. During the winter months, hemlock is an important food source for rabbits, snow shoe hare and squirrels, and if twig tips are littered on the snow beneath the canopy or irregular patches are chewed down to the wood on the upper branches, it is often a sign of porcupine feeding.

I like to think that a tree has four lives. The first is a young tree that struggles to survive and reach maturity. The second is a mature tree that finds its place in the canopy and supplies seed for the next generation. Dying and fallen trees provide the third and fourth lives and afford considerable eco-function in the forest habitat. Aging hemlocks become full of insects, which are dined upon by woodpeckers and other bird species.

When a large hemlock tree falls, it decays rapidly, creating spongy, damp soils ideal for seedling growth. These dead trees add additional moisture, keeping the forest cool and damp, and provide supplementary nutrients for other plant species. The rotting wood also creates habitat for salamanders and a variety of decomposers, as well as sites for ring-necked snakes to lay their eggs.

Culinary Uses

Young hemlock needles, simmered or steeped in hot water for a half hour, offer a pleasant tea. It is light in colour but very flavourful and can be enjoyed hot or over ice. This fragrant, warming tea was widely drunk among the Haudenosaunee (Iroquois) people and often sweetened with maple sugar. It was also a popular drink with the early settlers and was commonly served in Canadian hotels and inns during the 1800s. In the journal *Sketches of Upper Canada* written in 1821, John Howison documented, "Here I enjoyed all the comforts that are usually met within Canadian hotels and after supping on bread and hemlock tea, and supplying my horse with buck wheat and wild hay, I went to bed at an early hour."

I sometimes provide my guest a warming hemlock tea in fall or combine it with mint in summer to make a refreshing cold drink. I do find, however, that some get nervous when I reveal the source. Eastern hemlock is not to be confused with the unrelated poison hemlock (*Conium maculatum*), an herb in the parsley or carrot family found in moist areas. This extremely poisonous plant afforded the suicidal potion that killed Socrates.

Rich in Vitamin C

Like many conifers, hemlock is rich in Vitamin C. The needles were a common table tea of the Indigenous people, especially in winter, when their diet was largely restricted to dried foods. This beverage provided a source of nutrients to help these northern tribes get through the long, cold season.

Over the years, there has been some confusion as to which tree species was used by Jacques Cartier and his crew to help cure scurvy, a condition caused by lack of vitamin C. It was recorded that the Haudenosaunee (Iroquois) provided Cartier a tea made from the leaves of the "annedda" tree to help alleviate the symptoms of the disease. This name is similar to the Iroquoian word *onetda*, which means hemlock or evergreen, and it is possible that this tree may have saved the lives of these stranded voyagers. (Refer to white cedar for more information.)

Medicinal Uses

Offering a multitude of uses, hemlock truly lives up to the meaning of its scientific name *Tsuga*, which was derived from the Japanese words for tree (tsu) and mother (ga). Known as the "mother of trees," it has long been an important remedy for the Indigenous people of North America, and in the 1800s, the inner bark and "pix Canadensis" (hemlock pitch) were recorded in the *List of Canadian Medicines*. Some herbalists believe that hemlock from stream banks provides soothing medicine, while a more powerful remedy is obtained from trees growing on high, dry ridges.

It is the high tannin content in the bark and the volatile oils in the needles and pitch that are responsible for its medicinal effects. Herbalist Matthew Wood calls it a warming astringent, and it is used when stimulating, toning and drying qualities are needed. A tea or tincture is made from the fresh inner bark or needles, and an essential oil, obtained from distilling the leaves, bark or pitch, is known as "oil of hemlock."

Wounds

Hemlock bark contains rich amounts of natural tannins, providing astringent and antiseptic properties. An external wash made from the boiled inner bark helps reduce swelling and heal sores and burns. In addition, the finely powdered bark was applied to wounds, cuts and abrasions to stop the flow of blood. In some native languages, the tree's name translates into "sore-healing woman," which refers to these traditional uses.

Colds and Fevers

The aromatic oils in the needles have a clearing effect on the lungs and, when applied as a vapour rub or inhaled as an herbal steam, it eases congestion, croup, whooping cough and bronchitis. Due to the high vitamin C content and volatile oils, the tea, when slowly sipped with honey or maple syrup, is used as a remedy for colds and coughs. It is a classic ex pectorant, helping to open the lungs, relieve spasms and thin and loosen phlegm so that it is easily removed. Furthermore, its antimicrobial actions help fight germs, alleviate sore throats and combat general pulmonary infections.

Hemlock was esteemed as a nice warming herb for feverish conditions. In the *Trail Settlers Guide* (1855) it was noted that "a cup of hemlock tea, drunk quite warm in bed, is excellent, as well as sudorific."

Urinary and Digestive Systems

Oil of hemlock, rubbed over the kidneys, has a strengthening application to the lower back and kidney region, and tea made from the leaves helps warm a weak urinary tract that lacks heat. Moreover, when taken internally, its astringency was valued for easing diarrhoea, dysentery and abdominal pain.

Bones and Joints

Due to its warming properties, the diluted essential oil or infused leaf oil, applied externally, can strengthen the tendons and ligaments. Oil of hemlock also benefits knee pain, rheumatic discomfort, arthritis and other disorders initiated by cold, damp conditions that require a stimulating action.

Sleeping on Boughs

Travelers used the soft, fragrant boughs to cover shelters and sleep upon, to provide warmth and ensure a quiet, refreshing slumber. Not only did they offer comfort and invigoration, they also deodorized and disinfected, helping preserve one's health in northern woods. In

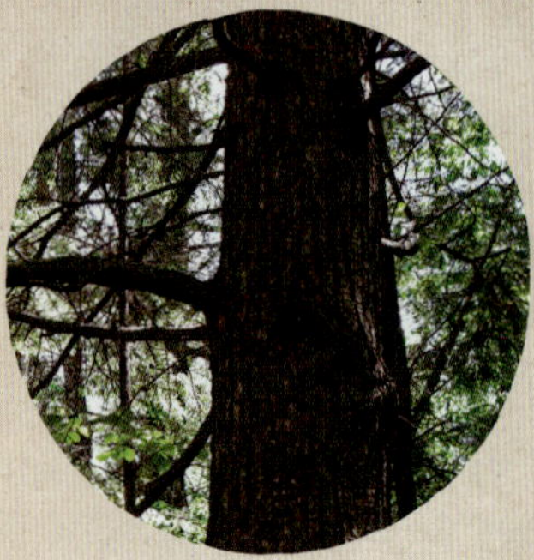

The bark was extensively used in the tanning industry

1892, Millspaugh wrote, "The stimulating effect of hemlock is well known and greatly utilized. A tired hunter arises fresh and invigorated from his bed of hemlock boughs."

Wood

While hemlock is a majestic tree of great magnitude, historically, it had little lumber value during colonial times. The wood is brittle, lacks durability when exposed to the elements and is subject to decay, cracking and splintering. As well, the dead branch stubs persist for many years, forming hard knots that dull axes and ruin saws, and for this reason was not highly sought after by sawmills. Despite this, hemlock is sometimes sawn into rough boards or planks for general construction, barn flooring, roof trellises, pallets and crates, and because it holds spikes and nails well, it was once used for railway ties after treating. It continues to be a source of pulp for paper and is now employed in the manufacturing of cellophane and rayon. Because the burning wood throws sparks, it ranks low as fuel and campfire wood, and hemlocks are not used in the Christmas tree industry since they readily shed their needles after cutting.

Tanning Industry

The deeply furrowed bark is a beautiful cinnamon-red colour with purplish layers and is so thick that it sometimes makes up 20 percent of the tree's cubic volume. Despite the fact that the timber was insignificant, hemlock trees were still heavily harvested in the nineteenth century, bringing in millions of dollars of revenue. Due to its high tannin content (up to 12%), the powdered bark was extensively used in the leather industry to tan hides and brought a good price from tanners. In the 1800s, old Canadian tanneries were built close to hemlock stands, where the trees were readily available. Once cut, large sheets of bark were peeled and piled to dry, while many bare logs were left in the woods to decay.

Hemlock still remains one of the chief sources of natural tannins for commercial tanning and is either used on its own or mixed with oak bark. Oak tanning produces a tighter grain, making leather less prone to breakage, whereas hemlock has a faster tanning time. Combining the two is thought to produce a better product than either on its own.

Other Uses

In addition to tanning, a decoction of the root and bark produces a mahogany dye which was used to colour spoons, spears, paddles and other wooden articles a deep reddish-brown. When mixed with alum, it provided settlers a good source of dye for wood, wool and cotton, a practice that lives on today in parts of the country.

The First Nations used the boughs to make primitive brooms and to line pits for storing corn, squash and other vegetables. Hunters sprinkled powdered hemlock bark on their bodies to mask their scent while hunting, and it was put into shoes to ease tender feet.

Cones of conifer trees have long been a symbol of female fertility. Hemlock's small cones were once dropped into green wax, strung into necklaces and worn by women who wished to become pregnant.

Lessons of Hemlock

Hemlocks can survive hundreds of years, and the tree's grandmother spirit and grounding energy can be felt as soon as you approach her. She readily shares her wisdom with any who are respectful; guiding and reconnecting us with the natural world.

Like her strong, majestic branches and hard wood, she provides stability and inner strength, and her solitary lifestyle helps those seeking independence and tolerance. While walking in her shade, the temperatures are significantly cooler in the summer and warmer in the winter. Her feminine energy is both gentle and protective, which is clearly sensed by the animals of the forest, as they migrate to her; for, like the oak, she will always provide fortification and a safe haven the entire year. However, she is like a mother protecting her young, and, parallel to her trait of throwing sparks when burned, she is clearly a tree that should be revered.

Hemlock mother is slow growing and long lived, and when in her company the most important lesson she has to give is the gift of patience. Just as the young saplings will sit and wait many years for the light to shine on them, you too, with patience, will have your day in the sun.

Juniper or Red Cedar

Juniperus virginiana

Cedre Rouge, Red Juniper, Baton Rouge, Red Stick, Pencil Cedar, Graveyard Tree, Fire Tree, Gin Berry, Geneva, Broom Tree, Savin Tree and Hackmatack

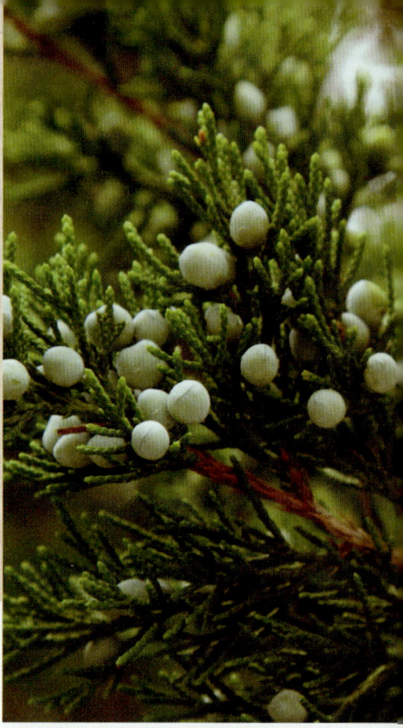

My first encounter with juniper did not leave fond memories. The leaves take the form of sharp, pointed needles, and, having approached too closely while young, I vividly recall the horrible prickles they carry. Lately, I've come to appreciate its many virtues and marvel at its rich history. Besides, without junipers, how would we flavour our gin?

Meeting Juniper

Although known as eastern red cedar, it is actually a juniper and not related to the true cedar (*Cedrus*) from the Middle East, as the name seemingly implies. It can rise to heights of a small tree, but usually reaches no more than nine meters (30 feet). It is slow growing. In fact, this tree is so leisurely at putting on stature it is known as "graveyard tree" because once it grows big enough to provide shade, it is time for you to depart this world.

The sharp pointed, scale-like leaves remain on the plant for five or six years before dropping to the ground. The foliage provides a lovely aromatic scent and can take on a purplish tint in the winter. Junipers are dioecious, meaning each individual plant produces either male or female flowers and both trees are needed to produce fruit. A small spherical ball can be found tucked among the prickly leaves, and strictly speaking, these "berries" are actually tiny, fleshy cones. When crushed, they release a pungent, highly resinous aroma. The fruit, which goes from green to bluish-black, is covered with a white, waxy bloom, and hangs on the branches two to three years before ripening. Therefore, it is not uncommon to see both the green, unripe fruit and the mature, dark purple berries growing simultaneously beside one another.

It seems that birds and junipers have an interesting relationship, both profiting from each other. When the fruit is eaten, the seeds benefit from the bird's intestinal flora. After passing through the digestive tract, the germination rate is three times higher than that of uneaten seeds.

Where They Grow

As a pioneer species, junipers are often one of the earliest woody plants to become established on abandoned sites. They grow unaccompanied in open territory, favouring dry, rocky areas, dunes and old fields. Because of their extreme hardiness, tolerating salt spray, cold, windy sites, and heat and drought, they have long been a symbol of longevity and strength. Their deep roots make them very sturdy, so they rarely blow over, and because they are securely anchored in the ground, they provide ecological benefits by holding eroding soil. However, these small trees are not able to tolerate shady conditions. Although there are records of very old junipers growing on exposed, barren sites, most have a short lifespan due to woodlands growing up around them. Another enemy that shortens their life is fire, and they will not become established or persist in areas frequently burned.

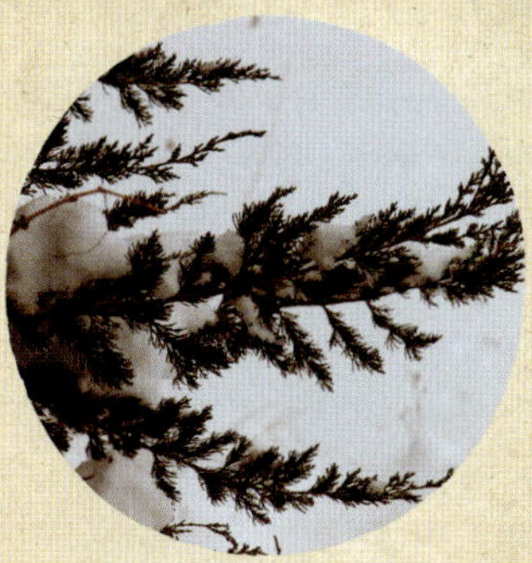

Junipers are extremely hardy

A Refuge for the Weak

Perhaps due to its habit of growing in harsh, open conditions, juniper was recognized for its protective presence and sheltering qualities, and became known as a "refuge for the weak." In the Old Testament of the Bible, it was juniper that concealed the prophet Elijah when he took flight from Queen Jezebel. It says in 1 Kings 19:4, "He went a day's journey into the wilderness and came and sat down under a juniper tree and prayed." A later story tells how Joseph and Mary, with their infant child Jesus, hid from

King Herod's soldiers beneath junipers when they fled into Egypt. Sprigs of juniper continue to be included in Christmas wreaths to symbolize juniper's important role in their escape.

Meaning of its Name

The name juniper likely came from *Juno*, whose root means "vital force." This origin may be due to its evergreen characteristic or the extreme hardiness that plants in this genus hold. *Juniperus virginiana* is called red juniper, red cedar, baton rouge and red stick, which describes its deep red heartwood, and it was dubbed "fire tree" in ancient times because when hot embers were covered with juniper ash, it was said to keep them alive for a week.

Wildlife Value

Junipers are valued by wildlife for the nourishment they provide and for the roosting and nesting cover they afford. The berries are relished by many birds, especially in winter, and it is estimated that 90 species, including mocking birds, blue birds, robins, wild turkeys and other game birds, periodically feed on them. Cedar waxwings are so fond of red cedar fruit that they were named after them. Part of their mating ritual is to pass a berry from one polite beak to the other until one finally decides it has its name on it. Other forms of wildlife, including opossums, chipmunks, red squirrels, mice, foxes, and skunks, also enjoy the berries. Due to the prickly foliage, most browsers find them unpalatable, although deer will nibble when hunger stressed.

Culinary Uses

It is said that eating juniper berries kept the body and soul together. The pungent fruit takes on a sweeter taste as it matures, and its culinary uses are many and varied. As far back as ancient Egypt, the dried berries were crushed or ground and used as a spice similar to pepper. By the fourteenth century, it was a well-known seasoning and commonly added to sauces and wild game in Sweden, England and Scotland to add a bitter, spicy flavour. In North America, Indigenous people cooked and mashed the fruit, then dried them into cakes for winter use or chewed a few berries to suppress hunger in times of famine. Today the ripe berries are ground as one would peppercorns and used in soups, stews, meat dishes, breads and cakes. It is best to use sparingly to avoid overpowering the dish. Two to four berries are all that is required.

The Making of Gin

If you have ever had a martini, you've had the pleasure of knowing juniper, for it is the aromatic berries that generate the distinct flavouring in gin. This is probably what juniper is best known for, and really, it was gin that made juniper famous. Of course, tonic raised the bar by joining gin and becoming a universal drink. It was felt that gin could brighten your life and was considered a "natural antidote to the emotionally debilitating effects of winter."

Despite the fact that during the eleventh century Italian monks used juniper berries to flavour their sprits, it was Holland that was recognized as the birthplace of gin. It was created in the sixteenth century by a Dutch professor of medicine, Dr. Franciscus Sylvius, who wanted to produce an inexpensive but useful diuretic remedy. He did this by mixing distilled juniper oil with grain alcohol and formed Holland's Geneva. The word "gin" didn't appear in print until 1714. It came from *genever*, the Dutch word for juniper. In the Scottish Highlands, bags of juniper berries were being collected and taken to markets in Aberdeen to be exported to Dutch distilleries. Gin soon found a following even when the diuretic properties were not required. In fact, it became so popular that people were becoming drunk and disorderly in the streets of England from consuming too much gin, and the authorities were encouraging the public to go back to drinking beer.

Medicinal Uses

Juniper berries are not just limited to the gin industry. At one time they were believed capable of "banishing anything injurious to the health" and restoring lost youth. Its earliest recorded medicinal use, as a cure for tapeworm, occurred on ancient Egyptian papyrus (paper made from reed growing along the Nile) dating back to 1500 BC.

Many of its healing qualities are due to its astringency and volatile oils, and for thousands of years it has been valued for its warming, stimulating and drying influences on the urinary system, circulation, digestion, lungs, uterus and lymphatics. Juniper is indicated for a cold, moist tissue state resulting in congestion, stagnation or constriction, and should be avoided in cases where the tissues are hot and irritable.

For medicine, collect the second-year berries in September or October, when they are fully ripe and deep, dark purple in colour. Dry them slowly for infusions or tincture them fresh. Due to its irritating actions, avoid using large or frequent doses when there is kidney inflammation, kidney failure, blood in the urine or large kidney stones, and because it can stimulate uterine contractions, juniper should be avoided when pregnant.

Urinary Tract

The volatile oils are responsible for juniper's diuretic action. It is more specifically classified as an irritating diuretic, because the aromatic oils irritate the membranes of the kidneys, causing an increase in fluid filtering, thereby provoking urine production and ultimately elimination. This stimulation can aggravate inflamed kidneys but proves very beneficial where there is chronic renal congestion or a depressed state of kidney function resulting in edema. The classic juniper person retains water in the upper arms, face, chin and lower part of the body, where the thighs are water-logged, causing a waddling gait, and the ankles and feet are swollen.

By alleviating sluggish conditions in the kidneys, juniper helps rid the body of metabolic waste and dissolve deposits in the urinary tract. When used in appropriate doses, it aids in the removal of accumulated gravel and mucus in the urine, and its antispasmodic effects dispel colic conditions that arise from these afflictions. Furthermore, the antiseptic influences from the volatile oils prove advantageous for treating urinary tract infections and cystitis. Conditions including diabetes insipidus (continual clear copious urine), deterioration of the ureter and incontinence can all benefit from juniper's toning action on the system.

Circulation

Culpeper claimed that juniper "provokes urine exceedingly and is a powerful remedy against dropsy (congestive heart failure)." Circulation burdened by edema caused by exhausted or congested kidneys can result in heart problems. Because juniper increases urine production, it can be part of the overall treatment for high blood pressure and congestive heart failure. It also stimulates the circulation to the extremities, alleviating cold hands and feet, and may help feeblemindedness and strengthen the brain.

For Muscles and Joints

Juniper's ability to restore lost youth was no doubt because of its effect on the muscles and joints. In ancient Rome, Pliny the Elder (23-79 AD) had considerable respect for Juniper's warming properties and its ability to relieve the aches and pains of arthritis, gout and rheumatism. Due to its diuretic properties, juniper assists in the removal of metabolic accumulations in the tissues and reduces inflammation in the joints. Additionally, the essential oils (oil of juniper), diluted in bath water or used topically in liniments or ointments, warm and relax the nerves, muscles and joints and aid in easing coldness of limbs, frozen shoulders, muscle spasms, strains, sciatica and muscular pain associated with poor peripheral circulation. In her book *Body in Balance: an Herbal Guide to Holistic Self-Care*, Maria Noel Groves suggests using an old folk remedy for arthritis where golden raisins are soaked in gin for 2 weeks and nine are taken each day for several months. Their anti-inflammatory and detoxing qualities improve joint mobility and relieve the pain from joint issues.

Digestion

Juniper acts on the mucosa of the digestive tract and is used when a warming and drying action is needed. It stimulates gastric juices and is specific for weak digestion and poor assimilation when there is sluggishness in the system or low digestive fires. Furthermore, its carminative and antispasmodic qualities from the volatile oils help to dispel wind in the stomach and bowels to relieve indigestion, bloating, flatulence, intestinal pain and colic.

Respiratory System

The volatile resins in the plant that vaporize on warm, summer days produce antiseptic compounds, and when breathed in are beneficial to the health of the respiratory system. North American Indigenous people poured a strong decoction of the leaves and berries over hot stones and inhaled the steam to relieve chest infections. It is now shown that the volatile oils act on the mucosa of the lungs and are an excellent remedy for excessive mucus and spasmodic conditions in the respiratory tract. A tea or tincture is used for congestion, asthma, coughs, colds, bronchitis, difficulty breathing and other cold, moist diseases of the lungs, and diluted juniper oil is inhaled or rubbed on the chest for pulmonary complaints.

Reproductive System

As a powerful emmenagogue that brings blood to the uterus, juniper has a warming, cleansing and strengthening influence on the reproductive system and aids a cold, damp uterus by easing cramping and encouraging menstruation. Because it stimulates uterine contractions, it was once given to women during labour to speed delivery.

However, the oil was also used for the purpose of aborting an unwanted pregnancy and was once known as the "bastard killer." In the Middle Ages, the phrase "to give birth under the savin tree (an old name for juniper)" meant to generate a juniper-induced miscarriage. Even as late as the twentieth century, Juno juniper pills, sold under the name "The Lady's Friend", were still available in European drug stores.

Adrenals and Diabetes

Having the ability to restore the adrenals, juniper is useful for chronic fatigue syndrome and recent studies have shown it helps lower blood sugar, suggesting a possible role in the treatment of insulin-dependent diabetes.

Skin Ailments

Historically, the inner bark was removed, placed it in warm water to soften, and employed as a bandage for open wounds. When applied externally, juniper's antiseptic action has proven to assist with sores, helping to prevent infection, stop bleeding and reduce swelling and inflammation. As well, a wash can be used for other skin conditions, including psoriasis, eczema and acne.

Protection from the Plague

In Medieval Europe, juniper was burned as a purifying herb during epidemics and plague outbreaks or strewn around homes to deodorize and cleanse the air affected by sickness and disease. During this same period, it was customary for doctors to hold a few berries in their mouths or chew six to ten per day when dealing with the sick to avoid being infected. This was believed to destroy harmful exhalations which sought to enter the practitioner.

As recently as the Second World War, essential oils were used in hospital rooms to fumigate them and prevent airborne infections from spreading. Lavender, thyme and juniper oils were found particularly effective. One amusing method of dispelling disease was reported in Scotland, where the house was fumigated with juniper smoke while its inhabitants were inside, after which the building was aired out and the occupants revived with whisky.

Disinfectant and Insecticide

Oil of juniper is an excellent disinfectant, and a few drops added to water can be used as a wash to clean walls, floors, bathroom sinks and kitchen counters. In the past, these same antiseptic qualities were also used to sterilize needles and bandages, and sutures made of catgut were soaked in a solution of juniper berries to hold their strength and sterilize them.

Cosmetic Preparations

The berries, wood and foliage are all steamed distilled to produce "cedar oil" or "oil of juniper" used in aromatherapy. In high demand by the perfume industry for its masculine, woodsy, fresh aroma, this essential oil is used to scent soaps, face creams, aftershave lotions, perfumes and other cosmetics. Combined with witch hazel and rosewater, it forms an antiseptic wash for acne and oily skin, or an antidandruff hair rinse.

Other Uses

At one time, the berries were dried on strings, smoked over fires and polished to make shiny black beads for necklaces. These were worn to ease the pain of rheumatism or suspended in homes to attract positive energy.

Red Cedar Wood

Although red cedar (*Juniperus virginiana*) is a small tree, the wood has been utilized for many centuries and is marketed as eastern red cedar or aromatic cedar. It is admired for its blood red colour, fragrant odor and resistance to decay. Of all woods, juniper is among the most durable, even when coming in contact with soil, and is able to withstand all types of weather conditions. It is the wood of choice for fence posts, and as a material for benches, it both endures the elements and has a very agreeable aroma when sat upon.

The red, easily worked wood is suitable for cabinets, furniture, carvings and small ornamental pieces; however, due to its scent, it is most famous for its role in lining closets and making cedar chests. The oils have insecticidal properties, helping protect clothes and woolens from moths. To renew the fragrance, simply sand the surface periodically.

Because there is no better material for making pencils, red cedar is also known as "pencil cedar." In fact, it was so highly sought after for this use that old fences were dismantled to reclaim the wood.

The burning wood emits minimal smoke. Because of its near absence, whisky stills hidden in the highlands of Scotland were fueled with juniper wood so that they would not attract attention from the local authorities.

Unlucky to Cut

In Wales, there was a widely held superstition that a person who cut down a juniper tree would die within a year. Because of this belief, it was customary to carefully preserve aged junipers and let them die of their own will. Similarly, other cultures considered it bad luck to destroy red cedar because it held the spirits of their ancestors. Thus, when a piece of the wood was worn around their neck, their ancestors would provide them protection.

The Naming of Baton Rouge, Louisiana

French Canadians called eastern red cedar *baton rouge*, meaning red stick, because the heartwood exhibited a vibrant red colour. When French Canadian explorer Pierre Le Moyne led an expedition in 1699 up the Mississippi River, they came upon red cedar trees stripped of their bark to reveal the deep red wood. Traditionally, these red wooden poles marked out the agreed boundaries of the hunting grounds between the Houma and Bayou Goula peoples. As a result of these red poles or sticks, when the state capital was developed on the site, the explorers applied the name Baton Rouge.

There is yet another large American city that was named after a native woodland forb. The Menominee tribe called the plains on the southern shores of Lake Michigan *shika'ko*, meaning "skunk's place." This area was aptly named, for at one time wild leeks (*Allium tricoccum*) grew abundantly across its range, producing a skunk-like odour. Skunk's Place, or Shika'ko, is now known as Chicago.

Protection and Purification

Since ancient times, this tree has been valued for its protective and purification powers. The wood was burned, not for its heat, but rather its fragrance. Juniper gives off minimal visible smoke; however, it is highly aromatic and for centuries was commonly used as incense in rituals and smudges to purify tem-

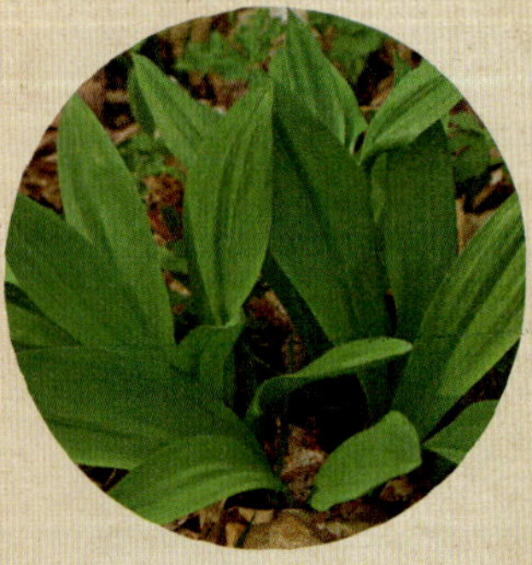

Wild leeks

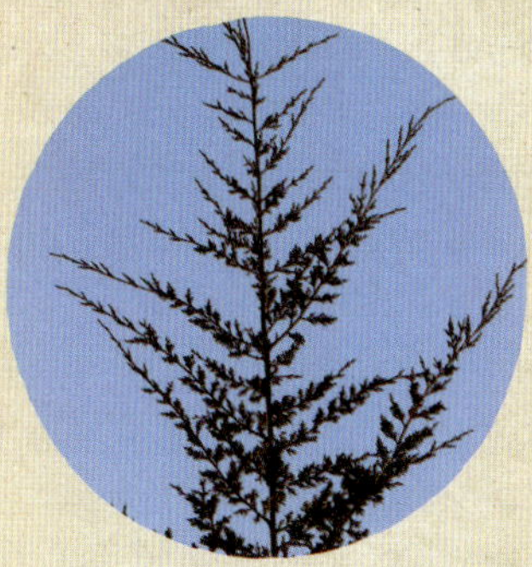

It was believed juniper could keep secrets, guard against theft and keep annoying visitors away

ples, consecrate homes, dedicate work spaces, welcome new familiars (pets) and bless babies.

Furthermore, North American Indigenous peoples burned it during their gatherings and used it in sweat lodges to emit its pleasant, cleansing scent. It was also used to produce "good luck smoke," especially for hunters, or the branches were hung in teepees to provide protection from storms.

Juniper was sometimes referred to as "broom tree" and mentioned in the Bible as such. Botanists speculate that this name may have come from the fact that juniper boughs were formed into brooms to sweep and cleanse temples. Like many strongly scented herbs, they were also hung in doorways or planted in gardens to protect against evil forces and spells, including banishing ghosts, sickness and bad luck. Wearing a sprig of the greenery protected the bearer against accidents and attacks from wild animals, and in Newfoundland, juniper wood was used to build fences and barns to keep out wolves and bears because it was believed they were repelled by the smell. Indeed, it was even rumoured that criminals once used it to mask their scent so dogs could not track them.

Theft and Annoying Visitors

At one time, it was strongly believed that junipers could keep secrets and guard against theft when grown by your door. If something was taken from you, *Frau Wachholder*, juniper's tree goblin, could be summoned to make the thieves return the stolen goods to their rightful owner. Often a juniper branch was bent and tied to the ground, and once the robber returned the stolen property, the branch was released.

In the Middles Ages, it was also customary to plant junipers beside the front door to keep witches and annoying visitors from entering. One legend says that the only way a witch could pass across the threshold was to correctly count the number of tiny, needle-like leaves. This proved so frustrating the caller would soon admit defeat and leave.

Folklore

In the Scottish Highlands, juniper was burned in Samhain (Halloween) fires to help contact their ancestors that had moved on to the otherworld. Homes were also fumigated three days before Beltane (May 1) to welcome summer, and on the Eve of Beltane, livestock were driven through two fires made of juniper as a means to promote purification and fertility. Carrying smoldering juniper branches around barns and fields to protect crops and animals was another common practice.

Dreaming of gathering juniper berries denotes prosperity, the birth of a son or being honoured or recognized for some great achievement. Burning juniper is said to aid in psychic powers, and like that of pine, the sacred smoke was believed to help prayers rise into the heavens.

Lessons of Juniper

Having the ability to disperse negative thoughts and stuck energy, juniper brings harmony and peace into our lives. Not only does it give us refuge, it provides endurance and strength to persevere when feeling weak or vulnerable.

Oak

Quercus spp.

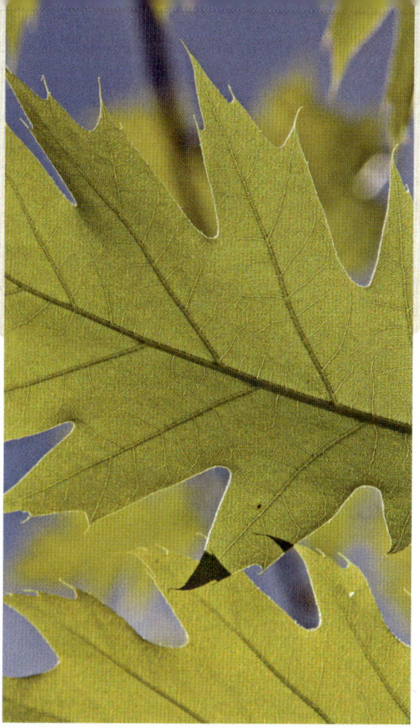

When Hudson came to North America in 1609, he wrote, "I sailed to the shore in one of their canoes ... the country is full of great and tall oakes." Oaks are so familiar to every culture that there is no other recorded designation. The botanical name *Quercus* is said to have been derived from the Celtic words *quer* and *cruz*, meaning "fine tree" or "a tree above all others," signifying their magnificence and splendour. They are noted for their slow, sure growth, as well as their massive size and long life. An old English saying, which portrays oak's leisurely growth habits, points out that "withy and sallow (willow) will buy a horse before oak will buy a saddle." Oaks also reach an enormous girth, and it is speculated that King Arthur's round table was made from a single cross-section of a large oak, which is still on display in Winchester, England.

Their life span differs depending on the species. Red oak (*Quercus rubra*) will only live a mere two to three hundred years but is relatively fast growing. On the other hand, the white oak (*Quercus alba*) may exist for five to six hundred years, outliving many other species in its community. As they age, they show knotted, twisted limbs that have withstood years of continuous ice and wind storms. Moreover, at Windsor Castle, some English oaks (*Quercus robur*) have been estimated to be over 1000 years old. An old expression says that an oak "takes 300 years of growing, 300 years of living and 300 years of slow decline." A lot can happen in 900 years. Just imagine what one of these old trees has seen in its lifetime.

King Charles and Royal Oak Day

For many years, oak has dominated England's forests and became a symbol of Britain's secure power.

Oak's strong, massive presence was naturally perceived to offer great protection and seen as a magical guardian. Held in high regard, it was associated with ancient kings and their ability to succeed in battles. However, these powerful trees also have a gentle, grandfatherly way to them, providing safety and shelter to birds, mammals and even kings. King Charlies II, who reigned the British Isles from 1660 to 1681, owed his life to the oak. He avoided being captured by Cromwell's soldiers after the battle of Worchester in 1651 by taking refuge in an oak tree. Upon his return to London to regain the throne, he adopted the oak as his emblem and declared "Royal Oak Day" on May 29.

Meeting Oak

In eastern Canada, two main groups of oaks exist. There are those in the red oak family, which have bristle-tipped leaf lobes and generally turn bright red in fall, giving this group its name. Some species associated with this category include red oak, pin oak (Quercus palustris) and black oak (Quercus velutina). Those with rounded leaf lobes are in the white oak group, to which white oak, burr oak (*Quercus macrocarpa*) and English oak belong.

The burr oak, when stripped of its leaves, is notorious for its gnarly appearance, which is reminiscent of the trees illustrated in front of haunted houses in a Hollywood horror show. This distorted look is due to their corky twigs. Because folklore proclaims that witches enjoyed dancing beneath the enormous branches, this image is very fitting.

The Nuts

Oaks have both male and female flowers on the same tree, which together produce nuts or acorns that are thin-shelled and nestled in a tiny cap. Oaks produce a bumper crop every three to five years. Many animals rely on oaks for food, and in return the regeneration of oak forests relies, in part, on the help of these forest critters. White oak acorns mature and drop in one growing season and are "sweeter" than red oak nuts. They do not store well and, once on the ground, either germinate or quickly rot. Because they are tastier, they are more apt to be directly consumed by mammals and birds. On the other hand, acorns on red oaks require two years to mature on the tree and need a stratification period to break dormancy. They store on the ground before germination and are often buried by animals as winter cache. Compared to white oaks, the tannin content in red oak nuts is higher; however, this compound is easily leached out, and buried acorns release some of their bitterness to make them more palatable.

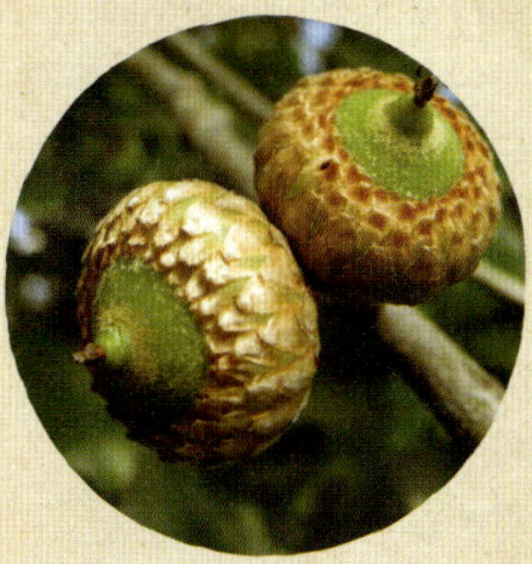

Acorns hold tiny caps

Oak Forests and Oak Savannahs

Oaks are commonly found in open savannahs or in mixed stands, enjoying the company of other deciduous trees. When Europeans first arrived in North America, they were marveled at the magnificent park-like landscapes of scattered oaks growing with a carpet of wildflowers. These cultural habitats are known as oak savannahs and were described as "a perfect Eden." Relics of aboriginal horticulture practices, they existed as a result of years of controlled burns. They are composed of prairie grasses and wildflowers with a scattering of fire-resistant oak trees. The custom of burning was widely applied by the First Nations people to maintain these open habitats as a source of game and to enhance the productivity of food plants such as berries and nuts.

Insect Life

The mighty oak is renowned for an extraordinary array of wildlife it supports, generously supplying food and shelter for a large number of insects, birds and mammals. More than any other tree, this keystone species is persistently used by insects. It is not only an important species for native caterpillars, they subsequently provide value to birds, which enjoy the protein-rich diet, especially to feed their young.

Oaks have a complex relationship with a family of small wasps called cynipids or gall wasps, which create swellings of various shapes and sizes on the leaves and twigs. A common gall found on oak twigs is the Oak Apple Gall. These galls are a rich source of tannins, making them a valuable resource for human use. Larvae feeding on the plant tissue stimulate abnormal cell development, resulting in round ball-like growth forming on the tree.

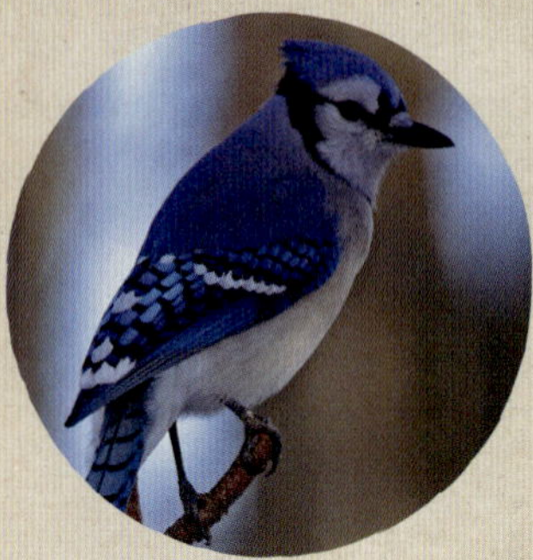

Blue jays help establish many oak forests

Wildlife Value

The benefits oaks provide in supporting and maintaining vertebrate populations cannot be overstated. In a good mast year, the nuts are highly valued, and competition is fierce. Deer, squirrels, raccoons and foxes are quite fond of them and black bears make tangle "bear nests" in trees while foraging. A number of bird species also utilize acorns, and frequent consumers include wild turkeys, ruffed grouse, ducks, woodpeckers, blue jays and crows.

Squirrels, nature's foresters, are attracted to the nuts and will either eat them on the spot or bury them for future use. Owing to the squirrel's poor memories, many nuts are forgotten and new trees are born. One would assume that squirrels are the main distributor of acorns; however, studies indicate that the majority of acorns are moved by jays. During acorn drop, blue jays can airlift more than 110 nuts per day and are instrumental in starting many oak forests. Gray jays are even more industrious, planting up to 140 nuts daily. Interestingly, acorns moved by jays have excellent germination, with a success rate of 88 percent. The explanation is that they generally select only viable seeds and reject any that are damaged. Thus, oak forests generated by jays are often of the highest genetic quality, being grown from the best seed.

Culinary Uses

Along with apples and hazelnuts, acorns were considered one of the three magical fruits and were said to satisfy all the needs of mankind. They were a staple in the diets of primitive people; so much so that oak was called "life giver." Pliny, of the first century, documented that acorns were roasted or dried and ground into nutritious flour to be made into bread. Across the ocean, acorns were also an important winter food in the diets of the Indigenous peoples, and in 1612, Captain John Smith noted, "In May and June they plant their fieldes and live mostly of acorns, walnuts and fish." Even successful agricultural tribes relied on the nuts, and

Indigenous women would store them in sacks for future use.

Most commonly used were the sweeter nuts of the white oak, but the bitter acorns of the red oak were also employed. The bitterness is due to the tannins within the nut, but these compounds are readily soluble in water and can easily be broken down and leached out. To eliminate the tannins, first remove the outer shell, then soak them in water for several days. This leaves a tasty, nutritious nut rich in protein, fat and carbohydrates. The time and number of rinses it takes to remove the bitterness entirely depends on the species of oak.

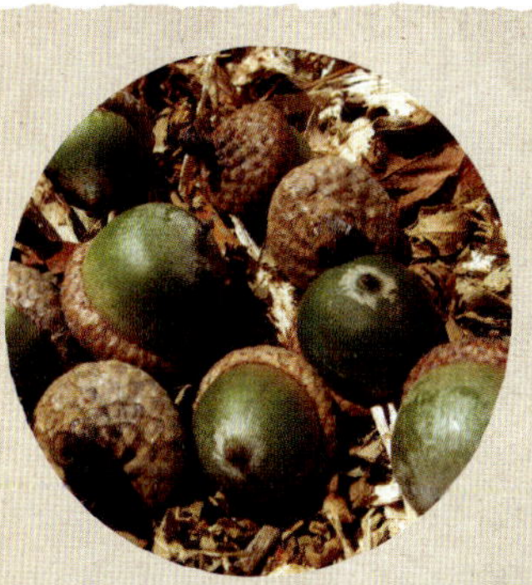

Acorns can be made into flour

Once striped of their tannins, they were roasted or laid in the sun to dry and then ground into meal or flour with a mortar and pestle. At this stage it was used as stew or soup thickener or made into hard, dry bread, by slowly baking it in primitive ovens. The early pioneers roasted the acorns and ate them as snacks, baked them in cookies, cakes and muffins or dipped them in sweet syrup to eat like candy. Today, few people bother with the slow process necessary to make acorn meal, but at one time this was common practice.

Similar to olives, the nuts were also placed in pickle brine to leach out the bitterness, and some species yielded good cooking oil. As well, roasted acorns were ground and brewed into a coffee-like drink, which some claim to be quite tasty. The beverage was commonly made when duties on coffee beans were high. In Europe, this drink, made from English oak, was known as *eichel kaffee*, or acorn coffee.

A Source of Mast for Pigs

Both domestic and wild pigs enjoy acorns and seem to thrive on them. In Medieval Europe, they were a valuable source of pig fodder, and in autumn farmers would set out their domestic pigs into oak forests to gorge on the nuts and fatten them up. In the seventh century, laws were made relating to the feeding of swine in woodlands (known as pawnage or pannage), and forested land was often measured in terms of the number of swine it could support. Early American settlers also realized acorns' worth for finishing hogs, claiming "the best ham grows on oak."

Medicinal Uses

The healing powers of oak were considered so great that simply walking around the tree and wishing the ailment to be carried off by the first bird that perches on its branches was thought to be an effective cure. In the time of Hippocrates, Dioscorides and Galen, English oak was recommended and frequently noted in old records. It is this oak that is considered "official" in Europe, whereas in North America the white oak is most commonly used.

Due to its high quantity of tannins, oak is naturally astringent, antiseptic and anti-inflammatory in action, and its medicinal application rests upon these qualities. It is the inner bark from young branches that is mainly used and is collected in winter or early spring, when the tannin content is highest. Its qualities are extracted by both water and alcohol and can be tinctured fresh or dry for decoctions. Because of its high astringency, large doses and prolonged use should be limited.

Tannins

The primary function of the tannins, at least from the tree's point of view, is for defense. Scientists believe this constituent acts as a chemical weapon against insect and fungal attacks, and increased production in the leaves and bark is closely linked with minimizing insect damage and other harmful issues. Oak bark is considered to be a very powerful and relatively pure astringent. Herbalist Michael Moore calls it the "basic astringent" and Matthew Wood regards it as the "model astringent," where others can be compared. For medicinal purposes, the tannins were usually taken from the bark, but in the early nineteenth century, Dr. Johann Rademacher removed them from the acorns through a distillation process, producing a product that he called *Quercus glandium spiritus*, or spirit of acorn.

The action tannins produce on tissues is characterized as astringent, and the taste related to this action results in a puckering or dry feeling in the mouth. Astringents effectively bind and tone tissues and reduce excessive discharge. They are specific for relaxed tissues that lack tone, are prolapsed, have broken down or exhibit extreme outflow of fluids. They are also used for their antiseptic properties to discourage pathogens.

Wounds

When it comes to wound healing, oak medicine freely provides astringent, antiseptic and anti-inflammatory properties. Not only do tannins help pull the edges of a wound together and staunch bleeding, they also kill bacteria and help create a barrier against infection by producing a temporary covering on the surface of the tissues. This protects the wound from further harm and infection, as well as hastening the healing process.

In 1791, Samuel Hahnemann wrote that oak bark is "the surest and most certain household remedy for gangrene." By toning the tissues and cleansing out putrid conditions and waste material, a compress or external wash is useful on cuts, sores, burns, bruises and wounds to check bleeding, decrease inflammation and guard against infection. It is recommended for weeping eczema, ulcers on legs, poison ivy, contact dermatitis in its early weeping stages, and other irritations of the skin. Furthermore, oak is employed both internally and externally to improve vein structure and strengthen the capillaries. It is particularly reputed for shrinking knobby, bluish-black varicose veins on the legs.

At one time, a tonic made from the boiled bark was applied to harness sores on horses, and the liniment was a "no fail cure" to relieve their sore, achy hips and shoulders.

Digestive System

Oak's astringent properties tighten and tone tissue in the gut and reduce inflammation and infection in the digestive tract. The constituents are carried to the gut lining to treat bowel problems, including lack of tone, leaky gut, internal bleeding and severe loss of fluids. This makes it valuable for ulceration of the bowels, intestinal prolapses and to cool and shrink inflamed or bleeding hemorrhoids. Furthermore, one of oak's primary applications is to control diarrhea caused by irritation of the intestine, and it is considered a superlative remedy for dysentery, which can lead to serious dehydration. Again, it works to not only control excess secretion but also to decrease inflammation and infection. For acute diarrhea, take a decoction in small but frequent doses.

Respiratory System

The tannins in oak also work on the mucous membrane of the respiratory tract, toning and drying up sinus congestion, post-nasal drip and excess discharge in the lungs. A decoction of the bark was traditionally used to treat bronchial infection and the early stages of tuberculosis, and employed as a gargle it benefits sore throats, tonsillitis and swollen glands. At one time, inhaling the fine powder was considered beneficial for consumption, and tanners that worked with oak were known for being particularly immune to this disease.

Spleen and Kidneys

There are few remedies that benefit the spleen. Oak bark is specific for a painful or inflamed spleen and is frequently combined with cleavers to remedy all types of afflictions to this organ. The spleen is part of the lymphatic system, and when it is not working efficiently, stagnation of blood and lymph fluid may result. Oak is invaluable in spleen dropsy (about one-third of dropsy cases are related to the spleen) and is specific for chronic lymphedema, particularly when caused from the removal of the spleen or lymphatic glands.

Furthermore, oak aids a weak renal tract where there is an excessive loss of clear fluids due to the kidneys not concentrating the urine efficiently. It also assists a sluggish urinary system resulting in edema, especially from the waist down.

Healthy Gums and Mouth

This is an outstanding herb for maintaining healthy teeth and gums. It has a mineralizing or calcifying influence, making it useful for preventing and curing tooth decay. Moreover, its astringent properties help reduce inflammation, heal infection and strengthen gum tissue, rendering it beneficial for weak gums, loose teeth, mouth ulcerations, canker sores and bleeding and swollen gums. Use a bark tooth powder or an oak decoction in a mouth wash for gum and mouth disease.

Alcoholics

Oak was once a remedy for alcoholics, helping those struggling with their addiction to control their cravings. It was suited for tipplers or someone who took frequent nips. These people were never really drunk but never really free from its influence.

Flower essence

English oak (*Quercus robur*) is the oak Dr. Bach used for his flower essence. It is for those who continue to fight, but never succeed – "the mighty oak is broken down." It is well suited to a strongly disciplined person who, for years, is slowly broken down by longsuffering and disease; never giving in, but never really flourishing. It nurtures inner strength and patience for those who are made discouraged, disheartened or despondent by struggle.

Cosmetic Uses

In 1817, William Barton noted, "The young branches stripped of their bark and rubbed with their ends against the teeth, render them extremely white." A decoction or powder also helps to dry sweaty feet, and rain water found in a hollow oak stem was believed to fade freckles.

The Wood

The English oak is said to have built the British throne, and its species name *robur* comes from the same root as *robust* or *strength*. Oak's strong, durable and solid wood was of great economic importance, and indeed, the success of Britain's industry is often attributed to its oaks. The timbers not only built homes and cathedrals; they were particularly advantageous in ship building. Britain's world-famous Royal Navy fleet ruled the seas and did so originally by the grace of the English oak. The Mary Rose, pride of King Henry VIII, was constructed almost exclusively of oak, with an estimated 600 trees being cut to build her.

Due to its leisurely growth, the wood is practically indestructible and noted for its incredibly dense, strong and durable qualities. It was an excellent source of building material and a superior choice for bridges, barns, tool handles, and wagon beds. Pin oak (*Quercus palustris*), with its notoriously tough branches, was used to pin barn beams; thus, the origin of its name. Oak panel became the hallmark of prestigious residences, aiding to the further devastation of our oak forests. Glowing honey-brown when polished, the wood continues to be valued for furniture, cabinets, flooring and veneer, as well as by carvers and turners.

The wood is permeated with compounds that discourage fungi and significantly slow decomposition. This, along with the fact that it is moisture resistant and impermeable to water, made oak a popular choice for the construction of wooden barrels to store dry goods, sugar and molasses. White oak was also favoured for whiskey casks, beer kegs and barrels to store and age wine. The tannins in the wood inadvertently improve the durability and taste of the wine, and "oaked wine" is considered of the highest quality. Moreover, oak was the preferred wood for plank roads, constructed in the early nineteenth century prior to gravel roads, where sawn planks were spiked to parallel stringers for wagons to travel over.

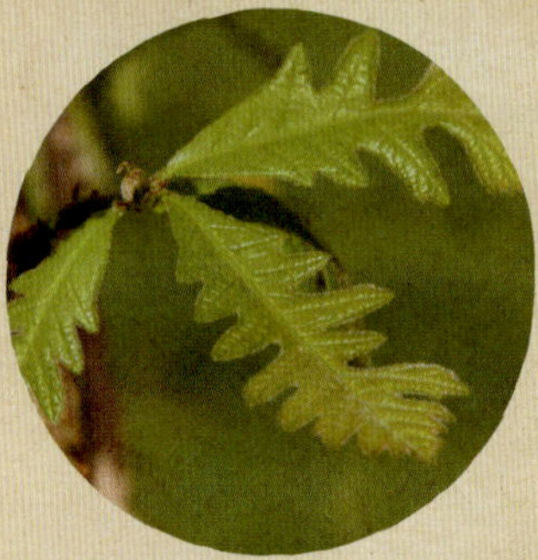

An acorn grows into the mighty oak to become the "king of the forest"

Oak was the classic wood for staves and wands, and for these magical tools the wood was cut during the waxing or full moon, after first receiving permission from the tree. Like hawthorns, it was believed that old oaks were the homes of fairies, and it was considered very bad luck to recklessly destroy one. If cutting was deemed necessary, it was customary to give the tree spirits three days' warning to allow them to vacate and find a new resident. Planting a new oak seedling was often recommended to help smooth the transition.

For heating homes, oak logs produce some of the hottest fires, as implied in this verse "oaken logs if dry and old, keep away the winter's cold." So warm were the fires, that burning oak in the hearth was thought to prevent winter illnesses or "draw off" sickness if a family member was ailing. From acorn caps, an excellent whistle can be created by placing the "cap" between your two thumbs along the flat section and blowing. The result is so loud it can be heard throughout the forest.

Tanning Hides

Tannins have been part of the leather-making process for centuries. Oak bark was used on a commercial level to tan hides and transform them into leather for shoes and saddles. Tanning procedures have changed little in the last 4000 years. The process involves treating raw pelts to render them resistant to water, heat and degradation by microorganisms. Other plant materials, including eastern hemlock, American chestnut (*Castanea dentata*) and staghorn sumac, were also valued by the tanning industry, but oak was so commonly used that it became known as "tanners' bark."

Dye

The most sought-after oak for dyeing was the black oak (*Quercus velutina*, formerly *Quercus tinctoria*), which was frequently called dyer's oak. The inner bark yields an excellent yellow pigment, known as quercitron, and proved to be one of the world's major vegetable dyes. It was once an important article of export to Europe and remained in commercial use as late as the 1940s.

Ink

Oak Apple Galls, produced by the gall wasp, contain two to three times more tannins than that found within the bark. These galls provide a strong black dye and, until the nineteenth century, were an essential ingredient in manufacturing high-quality ink. It is the tannins that help fix the pigment to the paper and prevent fading. It was not only used in classrooms; Van Gogh and Rembrandt drew with it, and many important treaties were signed with oak gall ink.

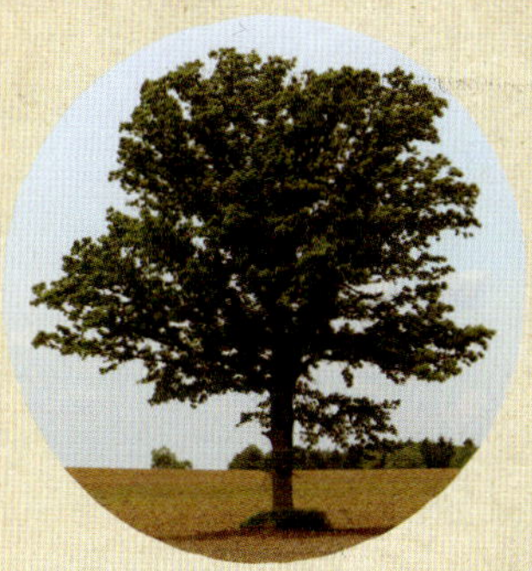

"Beware the oak, it draws the stroke"

The King of the Forest

The oak was associated with masculinity, and in the nineteenth century, gardener William Shenstone said that oak exhibits "the perfect image of manly character." Due to its extraordinary height and girth, solid branches and the fact that it can live many years, it was highly revered, especially in Northern Europe, and considered the "king of trees." It symbolized masculine qualities such as toughness, strength, steadfastness and endurance, and in his *Sylva,* John Evelyn called it the "pride and glory of the forest."

The sturdy branches rarely break in storms, and the deep tap root prevents it from toppling over. Moreover, it is one of the last trees to lose its foliage in fall, often retaining the dried, brown leaves into winter. These characteristics were thought to be signs of longevity and perseverance, and one only needed to carry a talisman of oak to gain access to its impressive qualities. As well, the Druids believed oak to be the tree of power and authority, imparting these virtues to any who stood within its shade.

The Tree of Thunder and Lightning

An old English saying, which may have some merit, states "beware the oak, it draws the stroke." This mighty tree seems to be prone to lightning strikes, and during an electrical storm it is best to avoid standing beneath its branches. There are a number of reasons for this heavenly flurry. Its thick, uneven bark and large open internal pores cause the wood to have low electrical resistance. As well, it is often found growing on the landscape in solitude and reaches great heights.

The Druids capitalized on this fact and regarded the oak as magical. It is surely no coincidence that they associated it with Thor, the god that has domain over rain, thunder and lightning. Due to the fact that oaks were frequently able to survive the blow of this fiery force and continue to flourish, they were sometimes considered the "life tree." Oaks that had been struck by lightning were known as "lightning oaks," and pieces of these trees were brought into homes to bring good luck, protect the occupants from "beings that would scare you at night" and guard against lightning strikes; the logic being that lightning never strikes in the same place twice. Baskets of acorns were also placed on window sills for the same purpose, and the Celts carved wands of oak to be used in weather magic.

Fertility, Abundance and Immortality

Since oaks were associated with rain making and the fertility of land depended on rainfall, the acorn also became symbolic of fertility and abundance. The tree was connected to Beltane (May 1); a celebration of Earth's fertility, mingled with the fertility dances of spring. On this day, the Oak King danced up and down streets decorated in oak and hawthorn leaves to petition the May Queen.

As a symbol of abundance, it was believed an acorn planted on the new moon would ensure money in the near future, and one carried in a pocket would bring financial prosperity. In ancient art, acorns were representative of male fertility and masculine vitality. Men once carried acorns to enhance their sexual attractiveness, increase male potency, preserve youthfulness and ensure long life.

Tree of the Sun

As it represents male energy, it only stands to reason that oak was also considered the "tree of the sun." Thus, it has an association with the Summer Solstice (Litha), which celebrates the sacred marriage of the sun god and the earth goddess. At this time, the sun's strength and power is at its height and personifies its ability to ripen the seeds of nature. While the holly king reigns over the waning half of the year, it is the Oak King who rules when it is waxing. At Midsummer, when the days begin to grow shorter, the Oak

King makes way for his dual self, the Holly King, but after midwinter (Yule) the Oak King once again defeats the forces of darkness and is reborn. He reveals himself as the vegetation god. It is not surprising that green men carved in wood and stone in Medieval churches most often displayed oak leaves.

To honour the sun god, the wood is used to fuel Midsummer fires. It was also customary to burn oak logs at Winter Solstice celebrations. This log was removed from the hearth before it was entirely consumed and reserved to kindle the Yule fire the following year. Acorns were also carried in the winter as comfort and reassurance that summer would return.

Tree of Hospitality and Generosity

The Celts were known for their generosity and took great pride in their hospitality. It was their custom to first entertain and share their food and drink before discussing business, and to welcome anyone seeking shelter. In the same way, oaks offer protection and hospitality without question or expectation, and the tree became an emblem of these qualities. Today, oak is still commonly used in names of inns, pubs, golf courses, malls and subdivisions, where hospitality and generosity are emphasized. Oak reminds us that compassion prevails when we have an open mind and generous spirit. We should welcome all those who require our assistance without prejudice and share what we have without resentment or reservations.

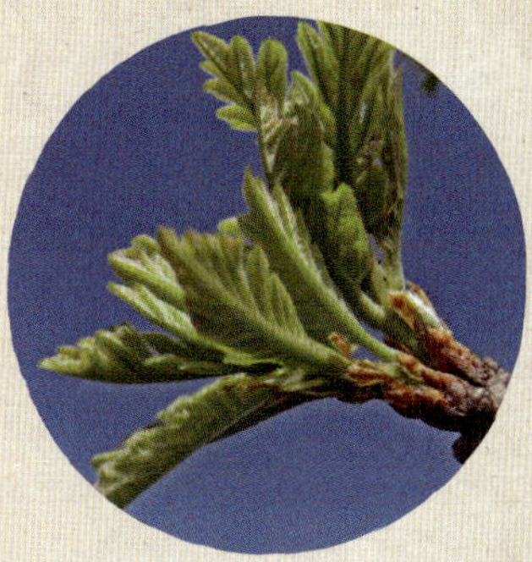

The tree of hospitality

Sacred Tree of the Druids

In Northern European cultures, the oldest sanctuaries were in woodlands. In sacred groves, trees were endowed with souls and considered to possess natural powers. For this reason, they were sung to, prayed to, and treated with great respect. Of all the sacred trees, oak is one of the most well-known. Over the centuries, they held deep religious and magical meaning and were highly honoured and admired in many cultures.

Oaks were held sacred among the Druids, who had mastered the art of intuition, knowing, healing and magic. They frequently met and worshiped beneath them and would only carry out their most sacred rituals and mystical ceremonies in oak groves. In the first century, Pliny the Elder wrote, "Druids never perform any of their rites except in the presence of a branch of it [oak]." The Celtic word for oak is *duir* and the name Druid was likely a Gaelic derivation that meant "people of the oak." Because of their association with oak groves, their dignitaries were known as "oak priests," and these people were considered to have "knowledge of the oak" or were "the wise ones of the oak woods."

Gospel Trees

In England, the term Gospel Oaks still exists in some counties. It refers to granting blessings beneath the shade of prominent oaks or the custom of walking around parish boundaries, a ceremony known as "beating the bounds," and reciting passages from the Gospel. At the time, property boundaries were often defined by oaks because of their long life and protective qualities. A verse written by Herrick mentioned such an oak. "Dearest, bury me under that holy oke or Gospel tree; where, though thou see'st not, thou may'st think upon me, when you yearly go'st procession."

To Communicate and Gain Wisdom

The Druids considered oaks to be a storehouse of wisdom and knowledge. The word *duir* gave rise to the Celtic name for oak and the word for door, both implying solidity and protection. This also suggested the oak stood as an opening to greater wisdom, enabling one to achieve inner strength and higher spirituality. It was viewed as a doorway between the worlds to gain access to spiritual guidance and a conduit to the truth. It was also perceived as a medium in which divine messages could be interpreted by man and these messages were said to be revealed through the rustling leaves or the wind whispering inside the hollow trunks.

The oak was not only a vehicle of heavenly wisdom for the Druids; it was also mentioned in the Bible for the same purpose. Judges 6:11-21 states that "an angel of the Lord sat under an oak tree at Ophrah and spoke to Gideon, telling him that he was to save Israel from the Midianites."

To stand under an oak is to gain power and strength from it; therefore, Merlin worked his magic in oak groves and used the top most branches for his wands. The Major Oak in Sherwood Forest, which grows near Edwinstowe, England, is thought to be about 800 years old. Beneath its branches, Robin Hood and his merry men planned their strategies of redistributing wealth. Treaty, council, witness and commemorative oaks are commonly marked and identified throughout Europe and North America to honour public declarations made beneath them, and they were common meeting places for village elders to decide on laws and morals.

Folklore

In Celtic folklore, the three primary trees of magic were oak, ash and thorn. Collectively they were considered the "sacred tree triad" and where all three grew together, one was likely to see the fairies dancing and playing. In Ireland, it is thought that fairies and other spirits lived not only in woodlands but resided in particular trees. As with hawthorns and elderberries, it is believed that the wee folk were particularly fond of ancient oaks, and the word *dryad*, an oak spirit or nymph, is defined as "those who delight in the oaks."

Bringing an acorn into the home would invoke kind spirits from the forest and improve communication with the fairy realm. Equal-arm crosses made of oak twigs (symbolic of the four directions, seasons and elements) were carried for protection and to safeguard against evil. In Ellen Dugan's book *Garden Witchery*, she states:

Oaken twigs and strings of red,
Deflects all harm, gossip and dread

Traditional weather lore states, "If acorns abound in September, snow will be deep in December." The oak is also consulted to determine when to plant seeds: "Sow corn when emerging oak leaves are the size of a squirrel's ear."

An acorn kept in the pocket would ward off rheumatism and other painful illnesses, and prevent the bearer from getting lost, both physically and mentally. It was believed that if you caught a falling oak leaf, you would have no colds all winter, and rubbing an oak trunk with the palm of your hand kept you healthy and strong.

To determine whether a couple will marry, drop two acorns in a bucket of water. If they float together, there will surely be a happy union.

Lessons of the Oak

Oak's noble and powerful presence gives us courage, strength and endurance to prevail against all odds, even overcoming seemingly impossible pursuits. Just as it can survive fire, ice and wind, it encourages us to endure, no matter what our challenges; helps us succeed in battles, including our own personal conflicts; and manifests our personal goals by providing a solid, sturdy foundation. It is for those who are discouraged or disheartened, taking the strain associated with worry, while nurturing inner strength, common sense and patience. It offers hospitality and protection without question, provides safety in its shelter and teaches us to be accepting, so that we have an open mind and a generous spirit.

Staghorn Sumac

Rhus typhina

Sumach, Vinegar Tree and Velvet Sumac

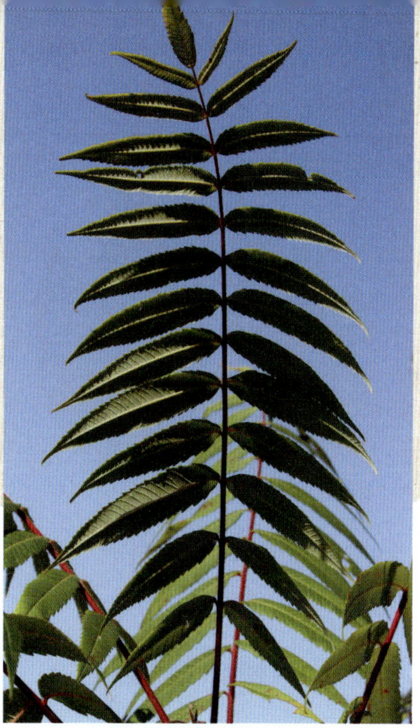

The merging crowns of sumac form a flat-topped canopy, creating a concealed open space beneath the branches. As kids, this protected spot allowed us to play hide and seek, build forts or observe passing wildlife. We could be found lying in the quiet shade, gazing at the clouds drifting across the blue sky, and in the evening, this became a magical place where we watched the flashing lights of fireflies.

Meeting Sumac

Staghorn sumac creates an outstanding show through the seasons and is cherished for its attractive fruit and beautiful autumn foliage. The large compound leaves are divided into toothed leaflets, giving the entire shrub a delicate, airy appearance. By fall, the foliage turns to glorious shades of orange and red, and it keeps its handsome spikes of scarlet berries throughout the winter.

Its beautiful, thick, antler-like branches are covered with velvety, soft hairs and possess orange piths. When broken, they exude a milky latex sap that was once put into hollow teeth to help eliminate the pain. The wood itself is inferior for campfires, as the burning twigs throw a great deal of sparks, giving the illusion of sparklers on a birthday cake.

Flowers and Fruit

The greenish-yellow flowers make a feeble display when compared to the erect fruiting clusters. These turn crimson by mid-summer, creating a striking contrast against the dark green leaves, and because they hold their shape and colour well, they are attractive in dried floral

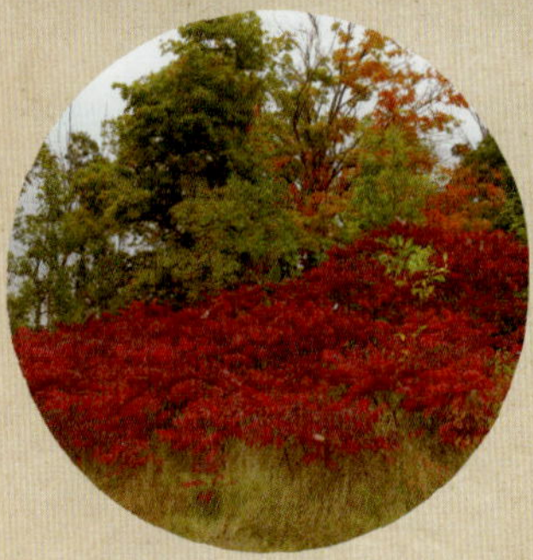

The foliage turns shades of orange and red in autumn

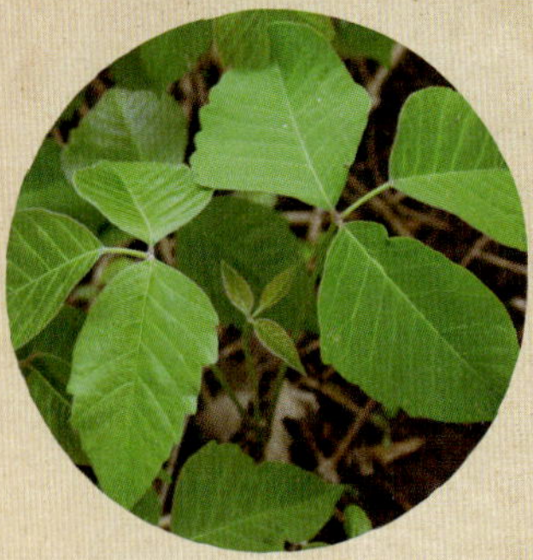

It is related to poison ivy

arrangements. The plush, cone-shaped fruiting candelabras, also known as bobs, contain a number of berries, each clothed in a reddish, hairy covering. The downy efflorescence is highly acidic, giving the fruit an extremely sour taste. Fading in colour by late fall, they become mined with insects and gradually crumble away the following spring. At one time, it was alleged that if you carried nine sumac berries in your pocket you would not be found guilty in court, or at least be served a lighter sentence.

Forming Clones

A solitary sumac is seldom seen, since this plant quickly spreads by underground rhizomes, forming dense thickets that can last several years. Through seed distribution, birds and mammals account for the establishment of new clones, and research has shown that sumac seeds that pass through the digestive system of animals germinate at a much higher rate than undigested seeds.

As a colonist, it is often one of the first shrubs to become established in meadows and transitional zones, slowly creeping out from forest edges. It thrives best in sunny locations and is unable to tolerate the shady environment of mature woodlots. It is also very drought-resistant and capable of growing in tough situations, making it valuable for dune stabilization or holding steep, gravelly banks. It seemingly wants to heal the earth, as it effectively prevents erosion and helps rebuild soils in disturbed waste areas. As civilization continues to degrade the environment, it is a blessing we have these plants that are eager to assist in restoring and protecting the earth.

Close Cousins

Staghorn sumac is considered non-toxic and quite safe, but it does have some less friendly relatives. The related poison ivy (*Toxicodendron radicans*) and poison sumac (*Toxicodendron vernix*) both produce white berries and contain urushiol oil, which causes a painful, itchy skin reaction in many. Sumac is in the *Anacardiaceae* or cashew family; thus, it is not surprising that another close relation is the cashew (*Anacardium occidentale*). Cashew drupes or "nuts" are located outside the fruit, dangling on the bottom. Like others in this family, cashews also contain a powerful oil irritant found in the lining surrounding the fruit, and when this shell is handled, a skin rash may result. For this reason, cashews are not sold in supermarkets with their shells intact. Fortunately, roasting at high temperatures destroys the toxic oils; thus, commercially sold nuts will not trigger a reaction. Urushiol oil is also present at varying concentrations in mangos and pistachios, which also belong in the cashew family.

Wildlife

Almost 100 bird species freely consume the berries, providing an emergency food source. The drupes persist through the winter, and early migrants returning in spring are particularly appreciative of the fruit when little else is available. Late in the season, the fruit clusters are also loaded with tunneling insects, which birds patiently pry out and eat. The red autumn foliage may serve as an evolved relationship known as "foliar fruit flagging." Both the plants and wildlife gain from this relationship. The brilliant leaf colour attracts the birds to the berries, and when consumed, they assist the plant by dispersing the seeds in their droppings.

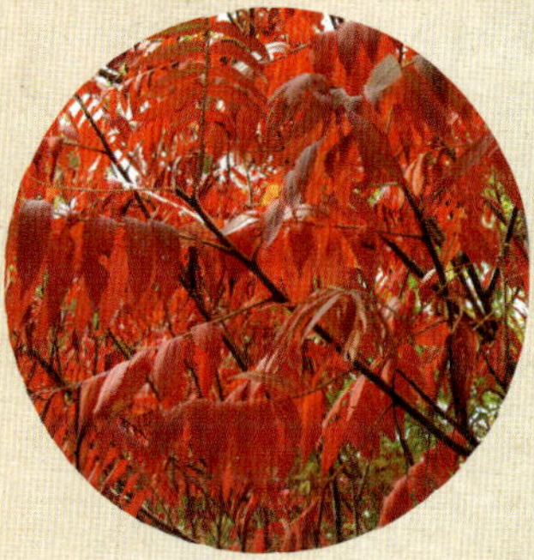

The bright, red leaves and fruit attract birds

The bark is a favourite food of cottontails, and many sumac trees are girdled during the winter months. However, the shrubs readily sucker back the following season, and biologists restoring habitats will sometimes plant sumac around the perimeter of newly established

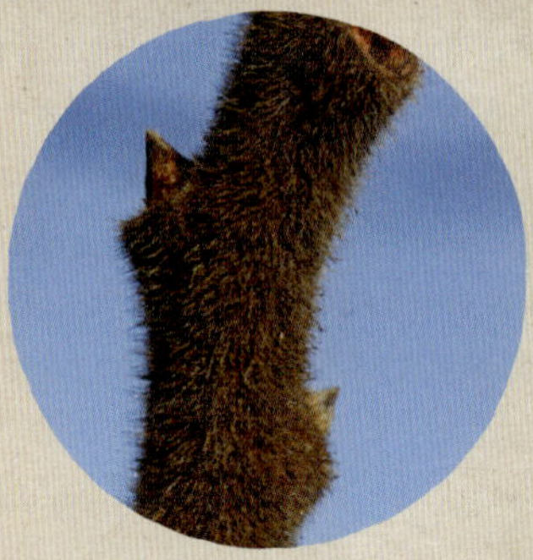

The fuzzy twigs resemble deer antlers in velvet

tree plantations as a sacrificial species, thereby protecting others from being gnawed on.

Some carpenter bee and wasp species hollow out chambers in the soft, decaying pith of dead sumac stems to lay their eggs. These insects then stock the chambers with paralyzed spiders and caterpillars so that they can be consumed by their newly hatched larvae.

Meaning of its Name

The antler-like branching and fuzzy twigs resemble a deer's antler in velvet, giving staghorn sumac its common name. The generic name *Rhus* was derived from the Greek word *rhu*, meaning to flow, and was perhaps given this designation due to its capability of stopping the flux of body fluids and hemorrhaging.

Sumac-Ade or Rhus Juice

Near Toronto, Ontario, 15 percent of the seeds recovered during an archeological dig were sumac, suggesting this plant was highly esteemed by the Indigenous people of the area. The crimson hairs that cover the seeds contain malic acid, giving the berry-like fruit a pleasant sour taste. By gathering the fruit soon after they turn red, a refreshing pink-coloured beverage similar to lemonade can be made and enjoyed on warm summer days. When chewed as a trail nibble, they leave a pleasant taste in the mouth and are said to relieve thirst.

Za'atar

Divers in the Middle East exploring ship wrecks from the eleventh century found quantities of sumac drupes. It was speculated that the berries were used for medicine, dye or as a spice. *Rhus coriaria*, a close relation, is widely used as a condiment in Middle Eastern cuisine, but staghorn sumac can be substituted with similar results. The acidic covering on the dried berries is used as a salt-and-vinegar type seasoning called za'atar, which is sold in many ethnic stores. There are regional differences in recipes, and traditionally each family would have their own secret blend; however, the common denominator seems to be oregano, thyme and salt, combined with sumac and sesame seed.

Medicinal Uses

Rafinesque (1783–1840) noted that sumac was a "good herb for all fluxes." Due to its cooling, astringent properties, it has proven to be a great remedy for preventing excessive fluid loss from any outlet, including the kidneys, bladder, bowels, lungs, uterus and skin. Herbalist Matthew Wood calls it the "leaky straw remedy" and indicates it when there is a "leak" somewhere in the system, causing drying of tissues elsewhere. The bark and berries are specific for debilitating fluid loss where the core is dried out, yet fluids are still being lost. High in tannins, sumac is also valued for its toning and restoring actions and is employed for conditions where the mucous membranes of the lungs, bladder and digestive tract are irritated or too relaxed. It is indicated for a weak, fragile person with poor immunity, anemic blood, inadequate bone marrow and inefficient kidneys.

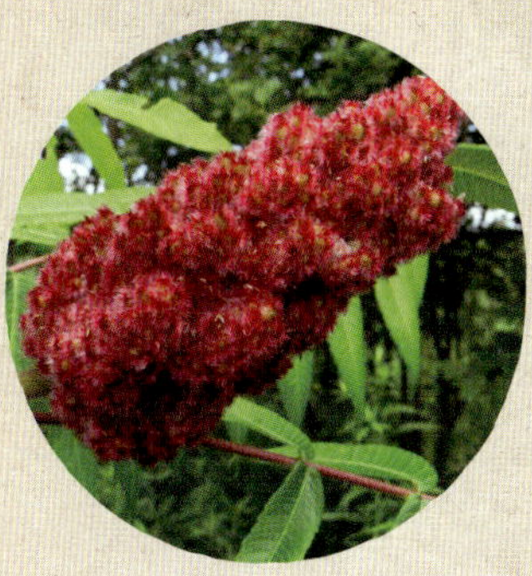

The fuzzy berries have a sour taste

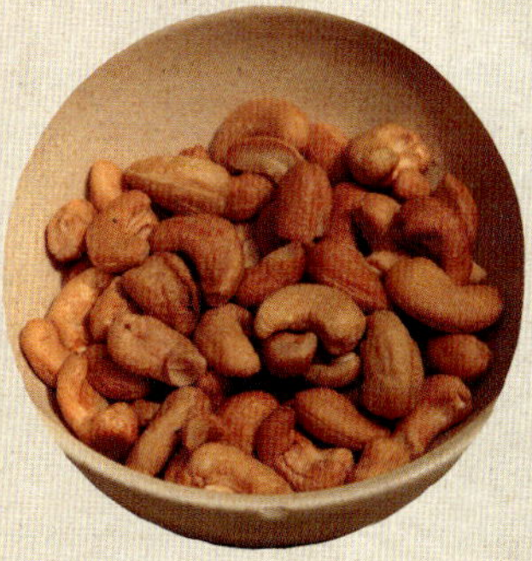

Sumac is in the cashew family

For it therapeutic actions, harvest the leaves through the summer months. The berries are gathered in early August as soon as they turn red, and are broken apart and cleaned to remove any insects. Dry the berries for tea or tincture them fresh. Heating releases the tannic acid, bringing out its astringency; whereas, a cold infusion releases greater quantities of malic acid and is more cooling in nature.

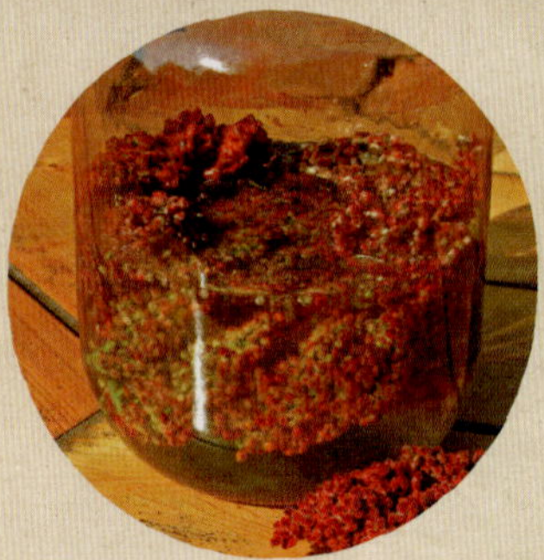

The berries can be made into a refreshing cold drink

Urinary Issues

Sumac reliably astringes, tones and strengthens the function of the kidneys. It is specific for weak, exhausted kidneys that are unable to efficiently move fluids, resulting in edema, or when the kidneys are incapable of retaining urine, causing a loss of fluids. It has gained the highest reputation for slowing excessive, frequent urination with the inability to fill the bladder before needing relief and to remedy dribbling or incontinence. In young and old, it can be taken before bed to help with bedwetting and the need to get up in the night. It also alleviates burning or painful urination and inflamed conditions in the urinary tract, whether caused from an infection or other issues. Furthermore, this remedy is reputed to help treat kidney anemia and low immunity. In this case the kidneys are not signalling the bone marrow to produce enough red blood cells due to renal insufficiency.

Diabetes

In London, Ontario, the noted Dr. Fredrick Banting, after conducting considerable research, found a cure for diabetes through his co-discovery of insulin. In his book *Banting's Miracle: The Discovery of Insulin* (1946), Seale Harris mentioned that Banting so greatly admired the Indigenous people that when he heard reports that they used sumac to successfully treat diabetes, he experimented with several bushels of leaves in an unsuccessful attempt to learn the secret of their reputed cure. This being said, sumac continues to be valued for treating type two diabetes and diabetes insipidus where a copious quantity of urine is passed with great thirst and excessive perspiration. It is believed to restore pancreas function and help keep blood sugars at a stable and more manageable level.

Toning Many Systems

Through sumac's powerful antioxidant and toning activities, it has the ability to improve cardiovascular and circulatory conditions. It is considered a mild heart tonic and may have a profound influence on lowering high blood pressure.

Furthermore, by astringing and decreasing inflammation of the blood vessels, it helps alleviate conditions like varicose veins, hemorrhoids, spider veins and fragile capillaries.

Sumac has toning and drying actions on the mucous membranes and is indicated for respiratory infections, colds, flus and allergies with copious, watery secretions from the lungs and sinuses. When these excessive fluids run down the throat, they overstimulate the cough reflex, resulting in a drippy, choking cough. Its cooling properties also prove helpful in reducing fevers, especially in children, and an astringent gargle is beneficial for soothing sore throats. Moreover, the tannins make it advantageous for toning the digestive tract, easing anything from mouth sores to bowel complaints. It is quick and effective at alleviating diarrhea and dysentery and improving inflamed conditions anywhere in the system.

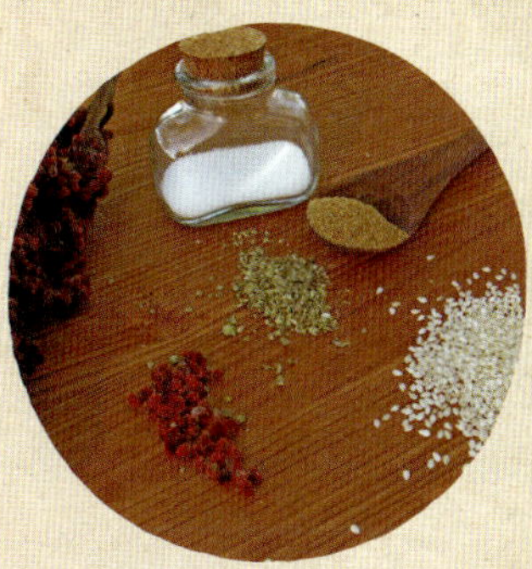

The fruit is made into a seasoning known as za'atar

Along with yarrow and shepherd's purse, sumac is commonly used to treat excessive menstrual flow, as well as flooding in menopausal women. It is particularly valued when profuse uterine bleeding is accompanied with a thin, water discharge. Through its toning and cooling actions, it helps clear damp heat in the reproductive system and benefits prolapsed uteruses.

Skin Complaints

The tannins present in sumac provide antiseptic and astringent qualities, and these actions make it valuable for a variety of skin complaints. A strong external wash or leaf poultice promotes tissue repair, reduces inflammation, slows bleeding and helps eliminate infection. Where its cousin poison ivy causes painful rashes, sumac can be applied to soothe skin irritations and other eruptions. It treats infected ulcers, wounds, sores, scrapes and abrasions, and speeds the healing of painful cold sores.

Tanning and Dyeing

Containing about 30 percent tannic acids, sumac's leaves, roots and bark were valued in the tanning industry. It was esteemed for gen-

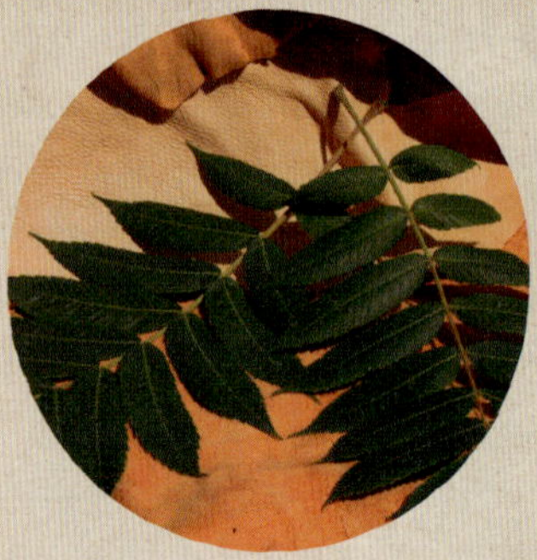

The leaves were commonly used in the tanning industry

erating fine leather that was flexible and light weight, and exhibited shades of light yellow or white. Through history, it was prized in the manufacturing of gloves, wallets, fancy shoes and book covers. Because American sumac has a higher percent of tannins than its European cousin (*Rhus coriaria*), it was much sought after. It rose rapidly in importance during the 1800s for manufacturing Morocco leather, and at the time large quantities were being supplied to the European market. The leaves were harvested in autumn when they were beginning to turn red, dried and milled into a fine power. By 1870 this product was being sold for $125 per ton.

After the American Civil War, a new industry was formed in the Southern states making use of sumac as dye material. Depending on the plant part and type of mordant used, the colours ranged from a rich to fawn yellow to solid black, grey, red or green. The mordant, usually tin, copper or an aluminous substance, added greater permanency to the dyes, and these colourants were unequalled for dyeing wool, cotton and silk. Sumac also afforded an excellent black ink. Care needed to be taken when shipping sumac with other goods such as marble. When the powder settled on white stone and became wet or even damp it penetrated it, staining it purple.

Other Uses

Oil of Rhus, extracted from the seeds, has a waxy-like consistency that could be made into candles or afforded oil for lamps. These candles burned brilliantly and are still popular in Japan, continuing a thousand-year-old tradition.

Sumac is a great utilitarian plant. The pithy center is easily removed and, like elderberry, was readily made into spigots for tapping maple trees. The hollowed stalks were made into pipe stems, and children fashioned them into blowguns. Although it never grows to a sizable diameter, the wood has a unique greenish sheen to it and is highly praised by wood workers for turning small items.

Lessons of Sumac

Sumac's umbrella-shaped canopy provides grounding and protective energy that conveys strength and stamina during periods of transition, so that you are able to generate confidence and self-assurance. Its healing influence also brings harmony to marriages and relationships and helps resolve difficulties.

Sugar Maple

Acer saccharum

Hard Maple, Rock Maple, Fire Maple and Bird's Eye Maple

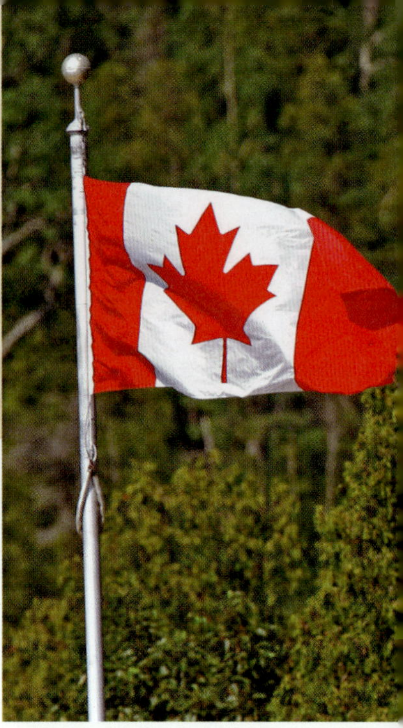

When young, often dessert at my grandmother's was simply a bowl of maple syrup. This may have been when I first fell in love with the maple tree. Its magic begins in early spring, when the sweet sap is made into syrup, and continues into autumn when it puts on a spectacular display of fall colours. The maple also holds a special place in my heart because it was my father's favourite tree. Due to its peaceful, friendly spirit, it is often considered the family tree. Its energy certainly fits my father's gentle personality and his love for family. He spent much of his time with his children and grandchildren. I can still see him lying in a hammock stretched between two enormous sugar maples beside the farm house with his grandchildren piled on top of him, telling stories and laughing. Afterwards, the mob would troop into the house to make ice cream sundaes smothered with maple syrup.

Meeting Sugar Maple

Few Canadians need an introduction to sugar maple. Even small children are able to recognize the leaf with five lobes that sits prominently on our flag. The botanical name *Acer* was most likely derived from a Latin word meaning "sharp," referring to the pointed leaves. Maples, like ash, prefer an opposite arrangement and hold their leaves across from each other. This ensures they are well exposed to the sunlight so they can soak up as many rays as possible. Most other trees, such as oaks, elms, cherries, hickories, basswood, birch and beech, assemble their leaves in an alternate layout.

This tree produces abundant seeds at two to five-year intervals.

The dried samaras, more commonly known as maple keys, produce two seeds, each equipped with a wing that resembles a helicopter blade. This design enables them to fly in the wind, carrying the seed a considerable distance from the parents. They germinate the following spring, easily penetrating the thick leaf litter on the forest floor. When young, we would stand on the picnic table and throw the keys into the air to watch them spin to the ground. Catching one as it fell was considered lucky, and a wish would be granted.

Climax Species

Along with American beech (*Fagus grandifolia*), sugar maple is a dominant species in climax, upland deciduous forests. The seedlings, being very shade-tolerant, can grow for many years under the shelter of others before reaching the sunny canopy. The cycle of succession slows when the forest reaches this climax stage. At this point, some type of a disturbance such as wind, disease or fire is needed to bring back species intolerant to shade. Not only does sugar maple dominate many Ontario forests, it was commonly planted in city parks and dubbed the "gentleman's tree." In the garden, sugar maple makes a wonderful shade tree, providing strong branches and striking fall colours.

The Friendly Tree

Sugar maples in a forest habitat grow straight and tall, leaving few lower branches. However, when found in an open area, such as along the roadside or in an old meadow, the lower branches remain, gracefully bending down to the ground and then swooping back towards the sky. This gives the illusion the tree is reaching down to you, evoking a friendly, peaceful atmosphere. This is fitting, as the sugar maple was designated our national tree in 1965, and the leaf is the emblem of Canada. In the late 1960s, the Canadian maple leaf also became a symbol of peace and love among the protesting hippies in the United States.

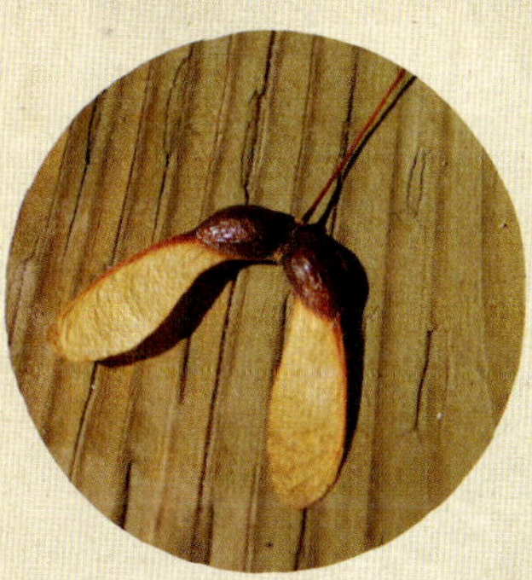

Maple seeds known as keys

Sometimes in woodlots, a few old maples can be observed dominating their surroundings. These large specimens are known as

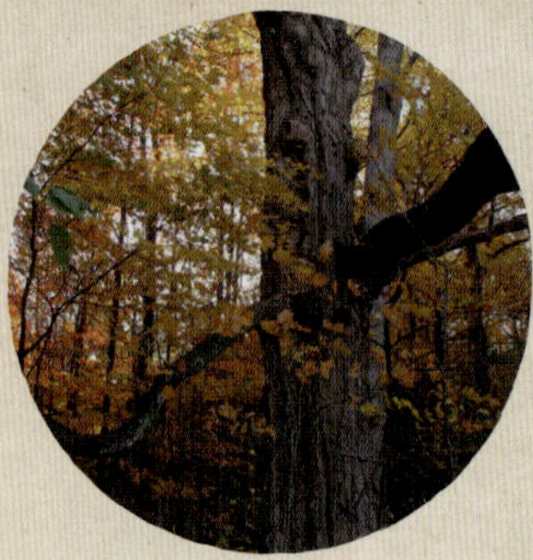

The branches reach down to the ground

below. Many also have a hollow interior, welcoming and sheltering the small animals in the forest and providing them a safe place to sleep and raise their young.

Fall Colours

Sometime dubbed "fire maple," sugar maple's dazzling fall colours of crimsons, oranges and yellows put on a vibrant display. With the

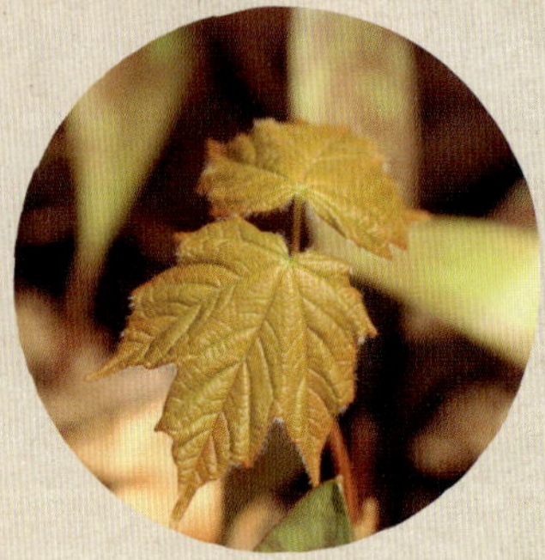

The seedlings are shade tolerant

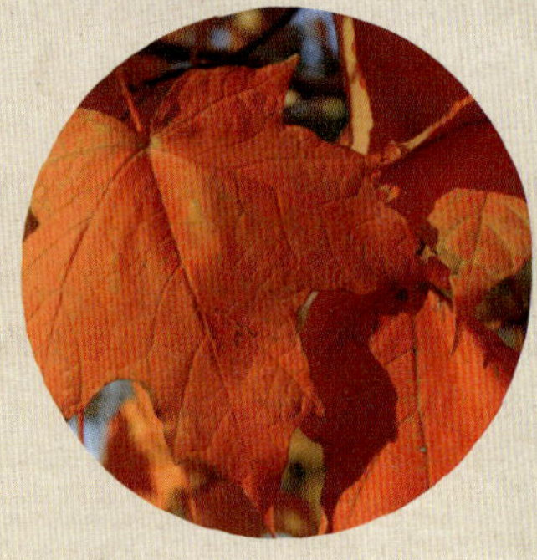

The leaves provide beautiful fall colours

"wolf trees." Like a lone wolf, they originally established themselves in an open environment and are much older than their adjacent neighbours. The absence of others has allowed them to grow large, wide-spreading crowns with heavy lower branches. Their evenly distributed limbs make them perfect climbing trees, greeting all those who want to be embraced in her canopy and look out at the world

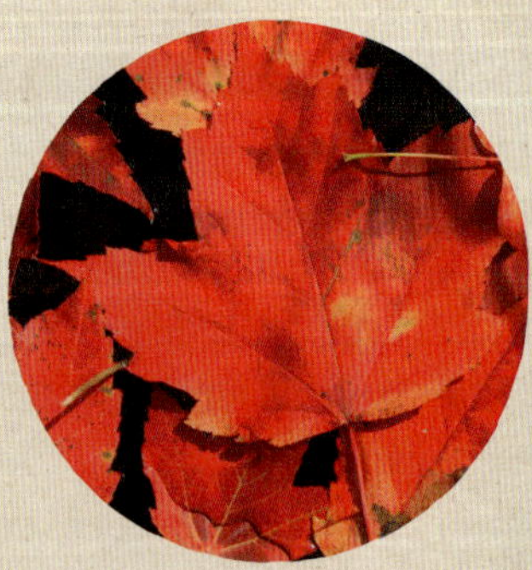

Red maple leaves turn red in the fall

decline of daylight and cooler temperatures in autumn, the green chlorophyll molecules in the leaf begin to break down and disperse. With the disappearance of the green, the previously hidden colours are revealed and a brilliant explosion of carotene pigment is unmasked. The rich, vivid hues attract thousands of leaf lookers to this part of the country. Depending on the year, the show lasts two or three spectacular weeks, until the wind finally blows them off their limbs. School children gather the leaves and press them between the pages of books to preserve their fleeting beauty.

Wildlife Value

Like people, wildlife species are fond of the sweet sap, and in early spring when things begin to stir, a multitude of activity centers around maple trees. A native woodpecker, known as the yellow-bellied sapsucker, drills evenly distributed horizontal lines around the trunk to start the flow of sap. After creating the holes, it returns at regular intervals to lick up the liquid and snatch up any insects that may have been attracted to the sweet substance. These, in turn, bring other insect-feeding birds looking for an easy meal. Ruby throated hummingbirds and some of our early spring butterflies, like mourning cloaks and tiger swallowtails, can be found visiting tree wounds to sip the sap.

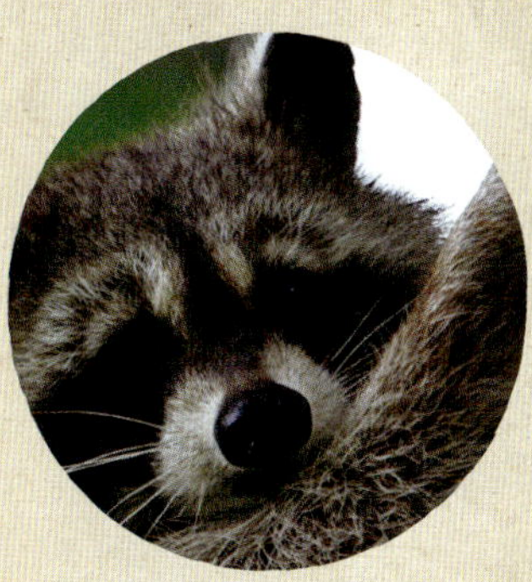

Old, hollow maples provide homes for wildlife

Where branches break off in storms, rot forms and cavities are created. These are enlarged by woodpeckers and chickadees, who then move in and raise their young. In subsequent years, these cavities are appealing to other forest birds and flying squirrels, who readily utilize them. As the rot continues to develop, the trunks become hollow. These trees are alluring to raccoons, where they rear their kits or use them as communal winter dwellings. We have such a tree in our yard, and we watch with interest each spring as the young peek out of the hole for the first time and crawl out onto the branches to explore their new world. Bats also use these ancient trees for roosting, both inside and under the ridges of the mature bark.

The Maple Nation

The Indigenous people in Ontario, Quebec and the northeastern United States consider themselves part of the "Maple Nation." Instead of political boundaries, ecological regions are defined by aspects that influence the daily traditions of the community, in particular diet. The native peoples of the Pacific Northwest belong to the "Salmon Nation"; those in the prairies are in the "Bison Nation." In the Maple Nation, sugar maples are considered sacred gifts from the Creator, and the sweet sap a blessing. Maples became known as the "family tree," as the people gather with their clan, young and old, to tap the trees. March is identified as the month of the "maple moon" or the "sugar moon," when Mother Earth starts to awaken and renew her gifts. Before tapping begins, ceremonies of thanksgiving are carried out to honour the trees and to thank her for sharing her offerings. During these celebrations, songs and dances are often performed to encourage a bountiful flow of sap.

Maple Syrup

The art of "sugaring" has been part of Canadian history for many centuries. The Indigenous peoples, and later the French Canadians and early homesteaders, knew about the sweet sap, and the making of maple syrup may be the most ancient custom in this region. Every year, trees are tapped in early spring and the sap is boiled down to produce nutritious syrup and sugar. The first sap in the spring was considered a tonic, and to this day the Indigenous people use it for this purpose. A great Wendat (Huron) chief said, "our maple water we drink 'tis sweet, well tasted, healthy and friendly to the stomach, whereas your wine and brandy destroy the natural heat, pall the stomach, inflame the blood, intoxicate and create a thousand disorders."

The Original Tappers

Probably one of the original "tappers" was the squirrel. They have an unmatched ability to source food and can be seen in the early spring nipping off maple twigs or gnawing on branches. Their tapping technique involves biting into the xylem to create a regular flow of sap that drips onto the bark, and when the water evaporates, it leaves a sweet deposit. They return regularly to joyfully gobble up the sugary treat.

Native Legends

How maple sugar was discovered is unclear. One legend says that a Haudenosaunee (Iroquois) chief pulled his tomahawk from a sugar maple tree, and when the weather turned warm, the sap flowed into a vessel near the trunk. His son, instead of going to the river to gather water as his mother requested, brought the sweet sap back to their camp. She used it to stew moose meat, which became sweet and delicious, and the sap has been used as a dietary staple ever since.

Another story says that when the Creator first made the world, maple syrup continuously ran from maple trees and one needed only to break off a branch for it to flow out as thick as honey. When Nanabozho walked through the world, he took note of those who were mindful and respectful of the offerings bequeathed to them and those who did not carry out the original instructions. When he came upon villages, he was dismayed to find that gardens were not tended, fishing nets were in disrepair and children were not being taught the traditional ways of life. Instead, he saw his people lying beneath the generous maple trees with open mouths, catching the thick, sweet syrup. They had become idle and lazy, taking for granted the gifts the Creator had given them. So he went to the river, dipped up many birch-bark buckets of water and poured them straight into the maple trees for a full moon cycle to dilute the syrup. Today, maple sap flows like water with only a trace of sweetness, to remind the people of both responsibility and possibility.

The Indigenous Method of Tapping

The First Nations people tapped the trees by cutting a diagonal notch in the bark with a tomahawk so that it sloped downward, and then drove in a long wood chip at the lower end of the opening in order to carry the water from the tree. The sap was gathered in wooden vessels known as *makuks* set beneath the dripping incision. These containers were constructed of birch or elm bark and stitched with spruce roots. Small quantities of sap were poured into troughs made of hollowed out logs, and hot rocks were repeatedly added to raise the temperature and start the natural evaporation. The sap slowly became syrup and then sugar. To speed up the procedure, the collected sap was allowed to freeze in shallow containers overnight and the top layer of ice was removed each morning, leaving a more concentrated sap. This was then boiled down in birch-bark kettles to make sugar. Once finished, it was stored in the same birch or elm makuks.

Tapping Methods of the Early Settlers

When the first Europeans arrived, they saw the Indigenous people making sugar from maple trees and were struck by it. Robert Beverley, who published *The History and Present of Virginia* in 1705, wrote, "The sugar-tree yields a kind of sap or juice, which by boiling is made into sugar. This juice is drawn out by wounding the trunk of the tree and placing a receiver under the wound ... it has been known among the Indians longer than any now living can remember." To the pioneers, for whom sugar was a rarity, it was love at first sight, and they quickly picked up the technique of sugaring to supplement their diet.

The art of syrup making has been handed down through the generations as part of our heritage, and over the years methods and equipment have improved. At the time of first settlement, the most common technique involved boring holes in the tree with an auger and inserting wooden spigots, often made from elderberry or sumac. The sap dripped into wooden buckets of basswood, which were collected with the help of horses and snowshoes. A further improvement was hanging the bucket from the tree a few inches below the spout, which was preferable to setting it on the ground and risking it tipping over. However, the most important advance in syrup making was the arrival and availability of metal. Metal spouts and buckets replaced wooden ones, and lids were fixed to the top of the pails to keep out dirt and rain. The sap was boiled in large iron kettles and later flat pans to speed the evaporation process.

Modern Techniques

Today syrup makers have turned to a network of plastic tubing as a method of sap collection and large evaporators to convert sap into syrup. It doesn't have the same nostalgic plinking sound you once heard from the old metal buckets, but it enables two people to run an operation that at one time would have been the work of twenty. Maple syrup making has become a lucrative business, and it is still common to find sugar shacks in local woodlots and maple products for sale in shops and grocery outlets. One thing that hasn't changed is that the making of syrup continues to be celebrated each year, and sticky-fingered children, young and old, still get out to enjoy pancakes and to welcome the return of spring.

Maple Sap

Sugar maple is the most frequently used tree to make syrup. Its sap offers the greatest concentration of sugar, ranging between 2 and 3 percent, although some claim that the less common black maple may afford a slightly higher percentage. The first sap of the year is usually considered the best, with the highest sugar content. It takes approximately 40 litres of sap to produce 1 litre of syrup, and at completion it is made up of about 63% sugar. Syrup can also be produced from red maple and silver maple; however, their sugar content is lower. Maples are not the only trees that produce sweet products. The sap from birch, butternut and hickory can also be made into syrup, but greater quantities are required and the quality is inferior.

Maple Products

Before refrigeration, maple sugar kept better and was easier to store than the syrup. Where maple trees were plentiful, it became the major available sweetener and a common medium of barter well into the nineteenth century. "Sugaring off," the continued boiling of the syrup, concentrated the sugars further to a point it granulated or solidified upon cooling. By slowly cooling and occasionally stirring the mixture, large sugar crystals form and harden into cakes known as "maple loaves." Today, these are often shaped into maple leaves and sold in gift shops as maple candy. If the mixture is rapidly cooled and beaten quickly, fine crystals disperse in a small amount of uncrystallized syrup, and a thick, creamy spread known as "maple butter" is produced. Maple sugar also makes excellent quality rum and cotton candy.

Maple syrup season is a festive time, and children look forward to it as they do Christmas. Spring celebrations are still held, and one popular custom is making "sugar on snow." The finished syrup is further boiled until it is foamy and slightly thicker; then the hot liquid is dribbled on clean, white snow in strips. Within seconds it cools and becomes chewy, like taffy. The lines are then twisted around a Popsicle stick for children young and old.

A custom adopted by European homesteaders was to sing to the maple trees and give some of the older trees a wee drink of whiskey or ale at Christmastide. This ancient tradition, known as "wassailing," was originally carried out on fruit trees, where the European people would sing and provide a drink to the trees to ensure a bountiful harvest.

A Northern Product

Canada generates about 80 percent of the world's supply of maple products. It is not the tree as such, but the northerly location that makes maple syrup production possible. Here, the appropriate climate in early spring encourages the sap to rise from the roots, bringing sweetness and nourishment to the tree as it starts to wake up. For this to occur, warm, sunny days (4 to 10 degrees Celsius) and cold, clear nights (-4 to -8 degrees Celsius) are required to persuade the sap to flow. Hamilton Percival wrote an account of ideal maple syrup weather in *Scribner's* monthly in 1904, saying, "The nights continue sharp and frosty, but the sun comes up with a smiling face and the wind is south and mild." Such weather typically transpires annually during February and March in Ontario, Quebec and the New England states and continues for about five or six weeks. Some old-timers say that the sap ceases to run when the first peepers (a frog species) are heard in spring. Although sugar maples have been introduced to other countries throughout the world, these areas don't have the right climatic conditions to produce the flow of sap, making maple products truly unique to Canada and the northeastern United States.

The Wood

Sugar maple has outstanding commercial importance. It not only sustains the maple syrup industry; it also contributes valuable wood products. Extensively used by cabinet makers and wood turners, it is crafted into fine furniture and bowls, especially where oak is scarce. It is particularly prized for Windsor bent chairs and in great demand for flooring and musical instruments. Noted for its strength and hardness, it was once fashioned into wooden runners for sleighs and now furnishes lanes in bowling alleys.

The white wood acquires a rosy tinge after being exposed to light and air, and the fine, close grain has a bright, satiny lustre, which is beautiful when polished. Occasionally, sugar maple wood can have a twisted, silvery grain filled with numerous little knots or eyes. Referred to as "bird's eye maple," this wood characteristic is greatly sought after for cabinet work and fetches a high price. Red maple lumber too can produce a distorted, undulated grain and is known as "curly maple."

Potash

At about 4 percent dry weight, sugar maple yields among the highest ash content of any wood, and from this, high quality potash was made. It was prepared by leaching water through maple ashes, and the liquid was then evaporated off in large iron kettles or pots, hence the name *potash*. This potash, also known as lye, was invaluable in the production of soap, which Great Britain required in large quantities for processing wool. It was also essential in the manufacturing of glass and gunpowder. To meet the demand during colonial times, large amounts were shipped back to Europe.

Because potash was in such high demand, the British government encouraged its production in America so that it could be exported back to England. It was dubbed the "black gold" of North America, and by the mid-1700s many acres of maple forests were routinely being cut and burned to yield additional income for homesteaders. This ended in 1807, when Thomas Jefferson's government passed an act forbidding the export of goods to the warring nations of France and Great Britain. When it became illegal to sell it in the United States, it was smuggled north across the border into Canada and then on to England. In Montreal, large "ash houses" survive as a historical reminder of this lucrative enterprise.

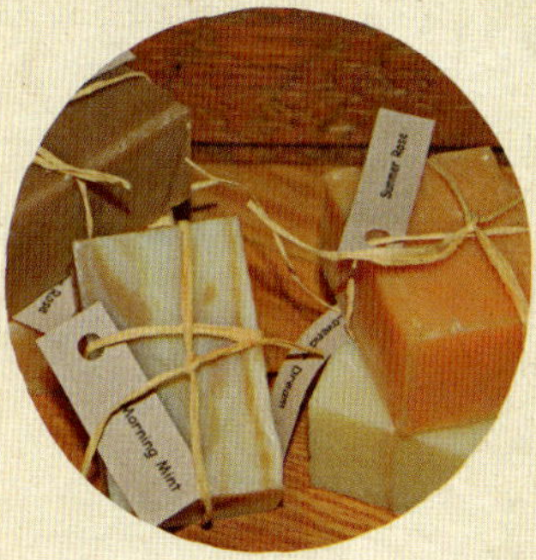

Lye, made from the ashes, make quality soap

Other Uses

The inner bark of the red maple, when boiled with copper, yields an intense black fluid. This afforded a good black ink commonly used in village schools in the early to mid-1800s. As well, the pioneers used it as a domestic dye to colour worsted and linen a lovely dark blue or purple.

Sugar Maple's Many Gifts

The word for sugar maple in several aboriginal languages translates to "the man's tree." This is very fitting considering all the gifts it has to offer the people. Besides its economic value of timber and sugar, it has been admired for its beauty and endless contributions to both the natural environment and villages. Maples are Canada's quiet leaders, giving

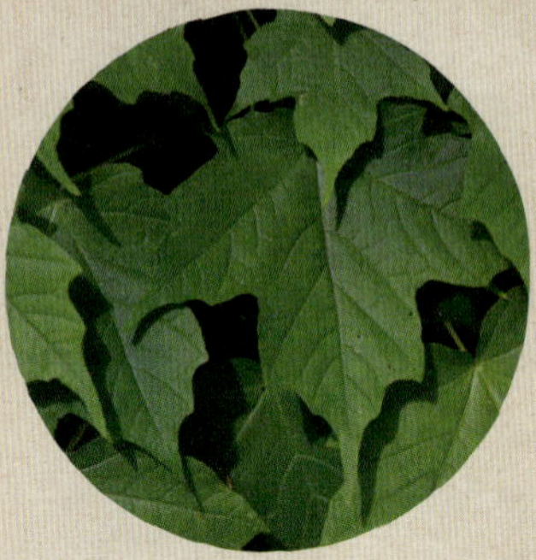

The maple provides many gifts

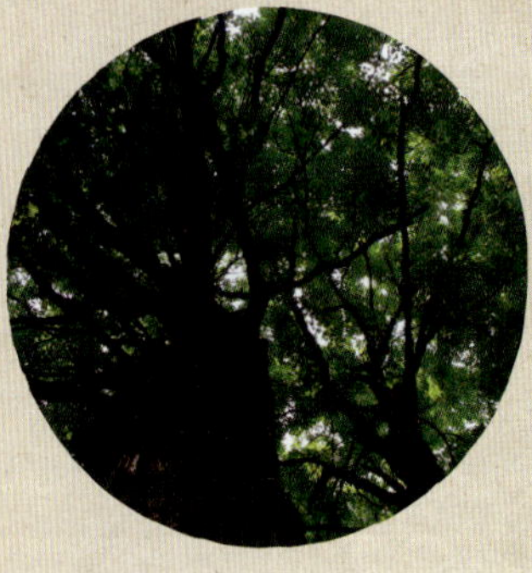

Maples are known as the "family tree"

all year and governing without being noticed. As stewards of the community, they continually take care of us and can be relied on to help maintain the well-being of society. We don't pay for these services; they are generously donated by the maple tree.

Maples contribute their wood to heat our homes in winter and provide syrup for pancake breakfasts that help raise money to support our local churches and volunteer fire departments. Thanks to their large canopies, they conserve energy by shading schools, homes and barns, and keep our livestock cool and healthy. By slowing the wind, they protect and hold soil in agricultural fields, buffer our water courses and reduce drifting snow on our highways. They run ecological services 365 days a year by purifying our water and air, not to mention providing oxygen and removing carbon dioxide from the atmosphere to be stored away. Centuries of fallen leaves have built up the soils on the forest floor to ensure a healthy environment for the next generation of seedlings, and every year the leaves that drop from our giant maples are tilled into gardens as compost.

Maples continue to serve on our civic beatification committee year after year, creating the crimson and orange colours in autumn to enhance both our rural and urban parks. The orange leaves that float to the ground are shuffled through or raked into piles, only to be jumped on and played in while we inhale their fragrance. Without being asked, they provide us shade as we picnic, read and receive company beneath their magnificent boughs, create habitat for songbirds, provide cover for wildlife and happily hold swings, tree forts and hammocks. This is a tree that just keeps on giving, and it is no wonder that Canadians have adopted it as their national tree.

Bride and Groom Trees

The sugar maple is known as the "family tree." For centuries, people have congregated under its canopy to make maple sugar and celebrate family events. There are many old photographs of homesteaders and their descendants assembled under such maples, which are prominently placed in front of their homes. Today we still gather under these friendly trees, benefiting from their peaceful, calming energy, generously enfolding families in their loving embrace.

In the early 1800s, it was customary to plant a pair of sugar maple trees on the south side of newly built homes so that in the summer the dense foliage would provide cooling shade to the building. Because homes were usually built when a couple got married, these trees became known as "bride and groom trees," as they commemorated a marriage and the start of a new family. These first homesteaders were not the beneficiaries of that shade, at least not as a young couple. They must have meant for their family to stay, to continue caring for the land and enjoying the trees planted with their wedding vows. I am so grateful for those who, 160 years ago, took the time to plant the maple trees around our old farm house so that my family and I can now enjoy the shade they offer. I feel as though I have a responsibility to these people for the gift they bestowed to me. I have no way of paying them back except to plant another sugar maple for the children that come after me.

Folklore

An interesting custom handed down through the generations is to pass an infant through the branches of the sugar maple to grant it a long and happy life. Carrying a twig is believed to bring success and abundance.

If silver maples turn their leaves to reveal their silver lining, it is said that they are showing their petticoats and a storm is brewing.

Because sugar maple is known as a "gentle tree," talking sticks were often made of the wood. In a traditional circle held by aboriginal councils, this stick was held by the person speaking so that they could express themselves without interruptions or judgment. In the same way, maple was sometimes used as a prayer twig.

Lessons of Maple

The sap of the maple tree runs between Imbolc (Groundhog Day) and the Spring Equinox (Ostara), and the leaves display their autumn finale between the Fall Equinox (Mabon) and Samhain (Halloween). It is not a coincidence that this tree's two major gifts occur around the equinoxes when the daylight is in balance. This tree can provide a sense of balance, as seen by its opposite configuration of branches and leaf arrangement, and sitting with maple can bring this attribute into your life.

Like the pentagram, which held magical association in the Celtic tradition, the five-pointed leaf offers symbolism: the four lower points venerate the four directions, elements and seasons, and the top point represents self. It is a reminder of the importance of honouring Mother Earth and ensuring her continuous care.

When people get busy, they lose touch with their inner peace. The energy of sugar maple brings calmness and serenity, creating a quiet peaceful place within and offering a fuller, more productive life. Maples also encourage creativity. Creative energy originates from a quiet place inside, allowing inspiration to flourish. It comes from our core when we feel calm and at peace with ourselves.

When our lives seem to be spinning out of control, like a key twirling in the wind, the maple reminds us to slow down and enjoy the path life has to offer. It allows us to admire the beauty and gifts Earth continuously provides; the deeper our appreciation for this beauty, the more gifts we will receive.

Trembling Aspen

Populus tremuloides

Enchanting Aspen, Quaking Aspen, Quiver Leaf, Quivering Tree, Shivering Tree, Talking Tree, Whispering Tree, Weather Tree, Shield Tree, Golden Poplar and Popple

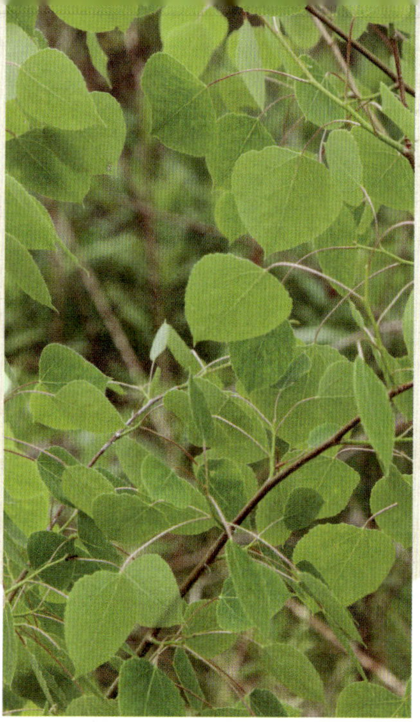

When I enter a stand of trembling aspens, I feel as though I'm walking into an enchanted land inhabited by faeries. The sunlight dappling through the leaves and the shimmering foliage dancing in the wind have a spellbinding effect that puts me in a joyful frame of mind. Aspen has an energetic spirit and is the tree of children, dancing, fairies and playfulness.

Meeting Trembling Aspen

Trembling aspen is noted for its rapid growth and resistance to inhospitable conditions. This pioneer species fronts the forest, often being the first to repopulate open areas and abandoned fields. It is a short-lived tree, maturing at 25, and by 50, exhaustion sets in and the heartwood begins to decay. Due to its intolerance to shade, it relies on major disturbances, such as fires or clear cuts, to provide lots of sunlight and the room it requires to grow. They are dominant features of early successional forests, but soon, more shade-tolerant species take hold in their dappled shade. They generously nurse the young trees that follow in their path. As these saplings grow, they slowly shade out the aspens, allowing the forest to succeed into the next stage of its life.

The Biggest Tree in the Woods

When hiking with children, I often ask them to search out the biggest tree in the forest. Invariably, they return to enthusiastically drag me off and present me with a large

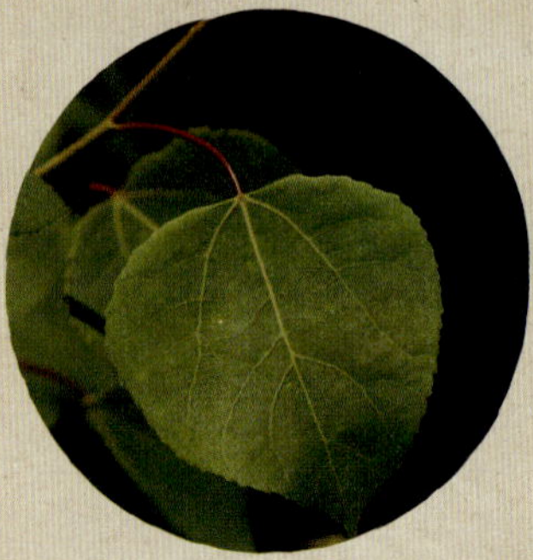

It does not tolerate shady conditions

beech, maple or oak. Although seemingly these are the largest trees, if poplars reside in the area, it is this species that wins the contest. Aspens are known for their ability to propagate through root sprouts and form extensive clones of many distinct stems. Consequently, a vast grove of trees, consisting of what appears to be individual specimens, are in fact a clone of trees, each arising from the same lateral root system. This adaptation is ideal for a species that dominates marginal lands. Because they are all part of the same organism and share a single root structure, they are all genetically alike and have identical characteristics. Therefore, while walking in an aspen stand you are actually passing through the biggest tree in the woods.

Stands of aspen form some of the largest organisms on earth. A clonal grouping, which originated from a single tree, may now include several thousand separate stems and cover many square hectares. As well, while individual stems begin to deteriorate around fifty years, the clone itself may well be among some of the oldest living organisms, reaching several thousand years in age.

Influences Affecting the Stands

Within an aspen grove, a number of relationships either prevent the stand from growing so thick that they eventually shade each other and deplete the population, or discourage other tree species from dominating the ecosystem to prevent stand decline. In western parts of Canada and United States, the pocket gopher, who lives mostly below ground, feeds on the roots of plants. In aspen stands they nip and detach aspen seedlings from the large network of roots, causing them to perish. Their tunneling and chewing allows only a few new shoots to grow, thus keeping the spacing such that new seedlings receive enough sunlight and adequate room to grow.

In higher altitudes, another deterrent to aspen regeneration is the suppression of fires. Even though the above-ground stems may die from the hot flames, the roots, which are often protected from the lethal temperatures, will sprout new trees soon after a fire moves through. Disturbances, such as the devastation of fires, are necessary ecological events in order for aspens to compete with conifer species. Aspens are soon replaced if there are long intervals without disruptions like fires.

An organism that quickly depletes aspen stands is the snowshoe hare, which counts aspen as one of its favorite foods. Hares nibble new growth until few seedlings are left. However, trembling aspens have evolved remarkable defenses against these browsing mammals. An attack triggers the plant to produce phenol compounds and terpenes, which are poisonous to hares. Usually the tree contains few poisons; however, high levels are found in new shoots that have been heavily clipped by hares in previous years. The poisons remain within the plant for two to three years, making the leaves bitter and less palatable. This deters further attack, reducing the amount of damage, and allows some protection to new seedlings.

Seeds

Male and female flowers emerge in early spring before the leaves make an appearance and occur in long, drooping catkins on separate trees. The seeds are equipped with tufts of silky hairs to facilitate their distribution by wind. Although aspens produce plenty of flowers and catkins, they seldom grow from seed. Pollination is often inhibited by the fact that individual trees produce either male or female flowers and large stands are usually all clones of the same sex. Even if fertilization is successful, the small seeds are only viable for a short time because they lack stored food and a protective coating; thus, aspens usually rely on vegetative methods to reproduce.

Geographical Range

Because trembling aspens can tolerate a wide variety of growing conditions, they boast the widest continental range of any native tree in North America and are found growing from Newfoundland to the Yukon and from the Canadian tree line to mountainous areas in northern Mexico.

The relatively smooth, greyish-white to green bark has a chalky appearance and from afar it is often confused with white birch. This light, reflective bark allows aspens to be well tailored to cold winter temperatures. This adaptation provides protection from sun scald, a condition that causes the bark to split from freezing and thawing in the winter sun. Another unique characteristic that allows aspens to thrive in cold environments is that the living bark of young trees contains chlorophyll and can carry out photosynthesis, a task usually reserved for leaves. By continuing to produce sugar for energy, this allows the tree a longer growing season when other deciduous trees are normally dormant.

The Quivering Leaves

The upper surface of the roundish leaves is bright green, while the bottom shows a silvery colour, making them reminiscent of silver dollars shimmering in the summer sun. It was once considered a sign that ominous weather was approaching when the foliage of trees turned over in the wind. Aspen was dubbed the "weather tree" because the light underside of the leaves shows their white lining or petticoat when rain is looming. By fall they turn a bright, buttery yellow. Lines in a poem written by Mandy Haggith depict aspen leaves in the fall:

One gold aspen coin
Woodland currency
For a priceless moment

Known for their excessive movement, the most distinguishing feature of aspens is the unceasing quivering of their leaves. They have action in their blood and seem to be constantly dancing to some bizarre, cosmic beat. Their continuous movement is due to the fact that the long, slender leafstalks or petioles, which grow at right angles to the blade, are flat, enabling the leaf to catch air currents. This feature causes thousands of tiny leaves to flutter and shake even in the slightest breeze, creating a distinctive rustling sound, as if being spattered by raindrops. This adaptation not only allows the leaf to twist easily, offering resistance from wind damage, it also improves photosynthetic rates by permitting more light through to the inner leaves. Furthermore, because both the lower and upper surfaces of aspen leaves are able to photosynthesize, the continuous movement exposes both sides so that more energy is generated for faster growth.

Aspen is often dubbed "noisy leaf." In the 1600s, a poem likened the constant fluttering of the leaves

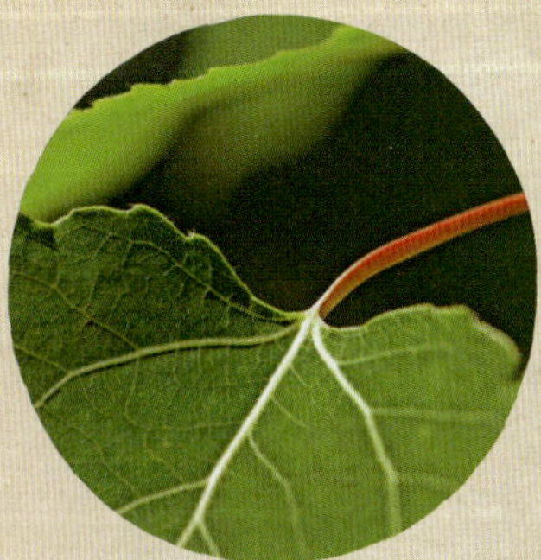

The leaf catches air currents, causing the leaves to quiver

to the tongue of malicious gossipers: "tongues that wave with every wind." However, it was also considered to be a magical tree, and placing an aspen leaf under your tongue was believed to make the bearer speak more eloquently.

Meaning of its Name

The genus name *Populus* may have been derived from two different sources. The Romans used the tree as sites of public meetings; thus, it was known as *arbour populi*, or the "people's tree." However, because of the incessant rustling and movement of the leaves, others claim that the name came from the Latin *papelin*, meaning "to babble." Many common names, such as quaking aspen, trembling aspen, quivering tree, shivering tree, talking tree and whispering tree reflect this characteristic, suggesting that aspen is continually on the move.

Wildlife Value

Trembling aspen is so generous with its gifts, it is said to feed no less than 500 species of mammals, birds, insects, fungi and other life forms. In early spring, the pollen is used by numerous native bees that are eagerly seeking a food source at this time of year. Many moth and butterfly caterpillars feed on the leaves and often defoliate entire branches. The foliage is not the only part of the tree utilized by these insects. The sap from wounds provides nourishment, and studies have shown that it imparts minerals to butterflies that afford them their unique colouring. This is not only necessary to attract a mate; it may also offer protection from predators.

In the winter months, ruffed grouse are often found foraging in aspen stands for both the catkins and buds, and their range closely coincides with that of this tree. Poplars often succumb to disease at 50 years, and their rotten stems provide excellent homes for cavity-nesting birds. Woodpeckers excavate nesting holes in the trunks and secondary cavity users exploit them the following year. Hairy woodpeckers utilize living trees, whereas the yellow-bellied sapsucker prefers trees infected with heart rot. Other songbirds use the cotton from the seeds for nesting material.

A number of other animals rely on aspen for food. The foliage and young branches are heavily browsed by deer, moose, caribou and elk year-round. In the spring, black bears climb the trees to eat the leaves, and during the winter, mice, voles, cottontails and snowshoe hares nibble at the bark, buds and twigs. Aspen catkins and foliage are the food of choice for porcupine. The terminal

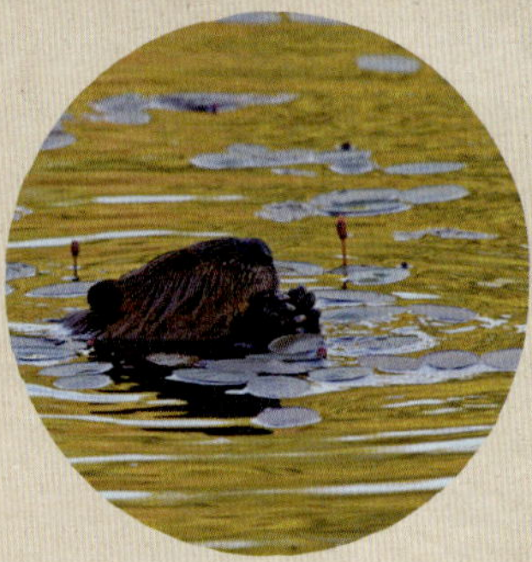

Beavers create ponds near aspens

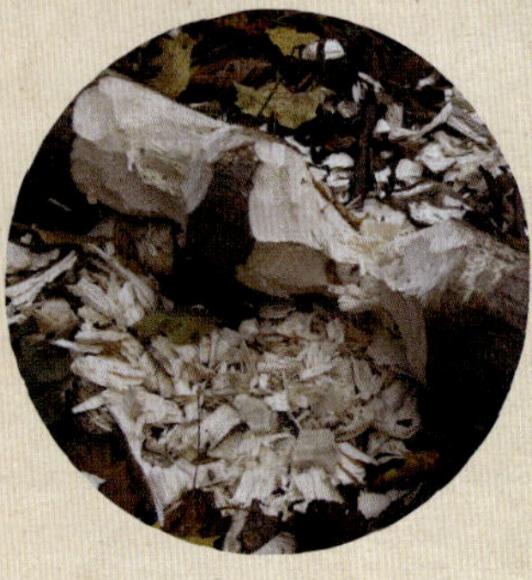

Beavers love aspen trees

branches are unable to support their weight, so they nip off the twig, eat the leaf blade, then drop the entire branch to the ground.

Probably the most enthusiastic users of aspen are beavers. The inner bark makes up the bulk of their diet, but the leaves, buds and twigs are also consumed. A beaver would never think of going into winter without a sufficient supply of food, and they take down a number of trees in fall to be stored at the bottom of ponds. However, nothing goes to waste, and the remaining wood is used to construct their dams and lodges. The depletion of poplar trees seems to be one of the main reasons a family of beavers will move to a new location. Their association is so prevalent, that during the time when beaver hats were the style, fur traders would seek out aspen stands to set their traps.

Medicinal Uses

Aspen, like willow, manufactures salicylates in its bitter bark. Salicin has chemical qualities similar to aspirin and is known for its analgesic (pain relieving) and anti-inflammatory effects. Its aspirin-like influences make it useful for systemic inflammation, fevers and to alleviate mild pain. It is effective for headaches, and Native American women brewed a tea to ease menstrual cramps. It can also be taken internally or applied externally for rheumatic and arthritic flare-ups, helping to relieve painful and swollen joints, muscles and tendons.

Traditionally, aspen bark was chiefly used to reduce intermittent fevers that would cause debility and weakness. By lowering an elevated core temperature and dropping it down to a normal range, it was valued for alternating chills and fevers due to colds, coughs and influenza. At one time it was taken to cure palsy, a form of paralysis accompanied by weakness and involuntary tremors; and ague, an illness involving fever and shivering (now often referred to as malaria, an infectious disease spread by mosquitoes). For these conditions, an early British folk remedy of interest was to pin a lock of the patient's hair to an aspen tree and tell them to recite the following verse: "Aspen tree, aspen tree, I prithee shiver and shake instead of me." It was then suggested to walk home in silence or risk breaking the spell, causing the cure to fail.

The tannins in the bark help to mend inflamed and slow-healing wounds by reducing the bleeding, relieving pain and stimulating the regrowth of damaged tissue. A wash is valuable for skin rashes and has excellent cosmetic benefits by toning and conditioning the skin.

The Wood

Several highland folk taboos, including those against using the wood for fishing gear, agricultural implements or in house construction, suggest that aspen may have been considered a tree of the fairies. Through the years, its uses to humanity have been limited. Today however, aspen is a major commercial product in the pulp industry and is generated into high-quality glossy paper for magazines and books. It is true that the soft, inferior wood is generally too weak for suitable construction material; nonetheless, when dried, it is lightweight and buoyant, making it ideal for household utensils, bowls, vegetable crates and boxes, wooden matches, oars and paddles. One unique feature of poplar wood is that it doesn't splinter. This has led to its use in playground equipment, wooden toys, sauna benches, surgical splints, tongue depressors, chopsticks and of course its important role as Popsicle sticks. Because it also shreds well, it is suitable as excelsior or packaging material to ship delicate fruits and vegetables, such as watermelons, cantaloupes and avocados, or to stuff furniture and coffins.

Because the leaves continuously shake, even seemingly without a breeze, it was believed that the aspen had a life of its own, and it was therefore never used for fire wood. It turns out that as fuel, aspen is of little value. As an English poet wrote, "poplar gives a bitter smoke; it fills your eyes and makes you choke." Due to the fact that it doesn't burn well and produces little heat it was often nicknamed "gopher wood," making it necessary to continuously "go for" more. One advantage of its poor burning characteristic is that floorboards of log cabins were sometimes made of aspen wood as a safety measure, to ensure a safe exit if the home should catch fire.

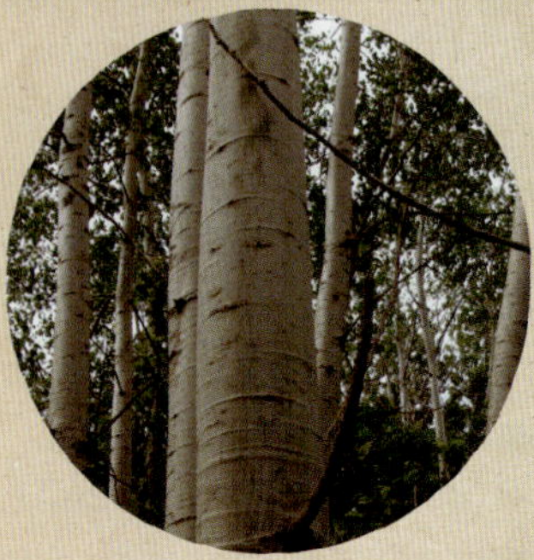

The wood was made into shields

The Shield Tree

Aspis is the Greek name for aspen, meaning shield. In Medieval times, the lightweight wood was indeed favoured among the Irish Celts for making shields, and the tree became known as the "shield tree." It was believed that the wood had magical powers that not only provided physical protection from the enemy but also guarded the bearer from psychic harm and darkness associated with fear. Due to aspen's magically protective nature, it became a popular choice to plant close to dwellings and buried treasure, to discourage thieves. Carrying a twig in your pocket also provided protection against theft.

The Trembling Tree

Many theories speculate as to why aspens rustle noisily. The Celts considered it a fairy tree and, sadly, trees that afforded such pagan respect often suffered ill fortune in Christian mythology. Here, they condemned this beautiful tree into something to fear and loathe. It was supposed that the poor aspen could never rest because the cross Christ was crucified on was made of its wood and it trembled in fear and shame. Even today, it is tradition in some areas to "dress down" or curse the tree while passing.

The Celts, however, had a completely different view. They believed the wind was associated with voices and was able to bring messages from God, ancient souls or spirits living in the woods. The quivering leaves were mediators that aided in communication between our world and the next, bringing messages from our ancestors.

Since aspen had a close relationship with the wind, it was considered sacred. It quivered incessantly because it was said to have the most acute hearing of all trees and was particularly sensitive to messages drifting through. In her book, *Tree Wisdom the Definitive Guide-*

book, Jacqueline Patterson noted that aspen "speaks of what it hears from afar." Even when there is no apparent breeze, they shimmer and move continuously in response to divine callings and should be listened to with an open heart. In the aspen, the wind finds a distinctive voice to inspire those who listen with patience and sensitivity, and it is held that if you pose a question and listen quietly, the tree will give you an answer. Moreover, as the wind passes through the leaves, its soft murmurs give visitors a sense of comfort and peace, and painters, poets and writers are said to become inspired under its boughs. In the past, aspens were also considered an important meditative aid, having a mesmerizing effect and encouraging a reflective frame of mind.

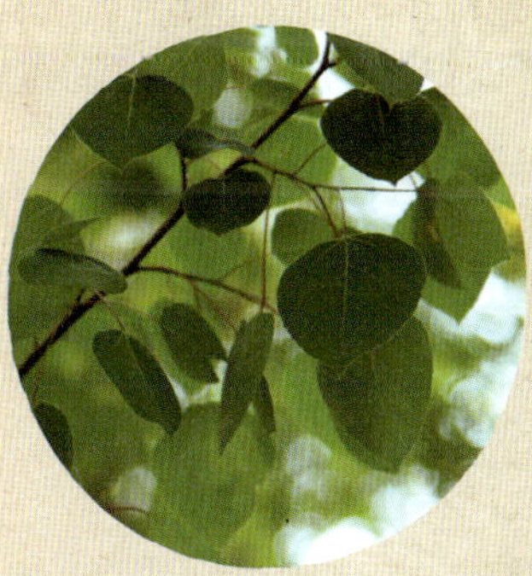

The beauty and uplifting energy of the aspen cheers the heart

Transcending Fear

In 1933, Franklin Roosevelt said that "the only thing we have to fear is fear itself." Fear has a way of creating and nurturing the demons within. The sheer beauty and uplifting energy of the aspen is enough to cheer any heart, and because it gives feelings of joy, it became known as the "tree that transcends fear." It is believed to ground and give strength to those who are nervous, have a fear of the unknown or have a fear of fear itself. In the *Victorian Language of Flowers*, aspen symbolizes lamentation and fear, and Doctor Bach used aspen's flower essence to quell deep fear and apprehensions. He noted that aspen helps us to understand that the power of love stands behind and overcomes all things. Once we know this to be true, we are beyond pain, suffering, care, worry, and fear, and we become participants in true joy.

Attracting the Fairies

Aspens like to stand apart from the crowd, away from other trees. Their flexible branches and energetic leaves are built to move. This spaciousness gives them the freedom to dance when the breeze begins to stir, and the fairies love to dance along with them. Over the years, many legends were told of people who, while standing under their boughs, disappeared into the land of fairies. Today, children collect poplar catkins and carefully put them in little saucers of water so that they can attract the faeries to their gardens at night.

Lessons of the Aspen

As a tree that sustains inhospitable conditions, aspen offers spiritual strength and endurance to face and overcome the fears and doubts that come with the unknown, and to confront the harsh realities that life presents us. It provides us a shield, offering qualities of resistance, perseverance, courage, fearlessness and inner power. Although aspens stand away from other trees, they grow together in groves, forming communities. This teaches us that we, too, are part of a community and should have compassion for those living around us, just as the aspen cares for and nurtures its neighbours.

Aspen's unceasing movement is a beautiful reminder of nature's constant presence and the sacred world around us. As the wind passes through the leaves, they continuously whisper messages. Listen within and find comfort in its voice.

Trembling aspens adore having children play beneath them. Their energetic, childlike spirit is like that of a tail-wagging puppy, teaching us that life has a playful side to it. Because of its lighthearted expression, to sit under an aspen encourages us to take life less seriously by looking at the world like a child again and participating in its true joy.

White Ash

Fraxinus americana

American Ash

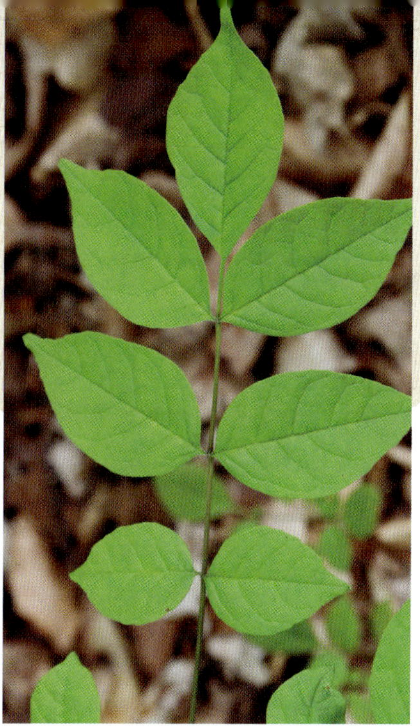

Among the Celts, ash was considered the "Great World Tree" or "Tree of Life," and it continues to be depicted on jewelry and other forms of art. In Norse mythology, this sacred tree, known as "Yggdrasil," was believed to support the entire universe. The original enchanted ash was very large, with its roots growing into the depths of the earth, its trunk reaching into the heavens and its boughs spreading over all the lands. It connected the heavens and the earth and formed a union between the gods, mankind and the spirit world. At its roots was the serpent, representing female earth energy, and in its crown sat the eagle, symbolizing the male energy of the sky. The squirrel ran up and down the tree, carrying messages between the serpent and eagle; and deer, where the great rivers flowed from its antlers, fed on the foliage. The leaves that fell were returned to the roots to nourish the tree, symbolic of the cycle of death and rebirth.

First Man Born of Ash

Central to the beliefs of many ancient cultures, ash was thought to be the tree from which the human race began. The Vikings thought that the first man was born from ash and that the ancient ash tree, Yggdrasill, held unborn souls in its limbs. Because of their great connection to this magical tree, the Vikings themselves were referred to as *Aescling*, meaning "men of ash." In Scandinavia, when the world was new, the original man was created from an ash tree, whereas the first woman was fashioned from an elm. After giving humans life and a soul, the god Odin called man Askir and woman Embla after their respective trees. However, in the highlands

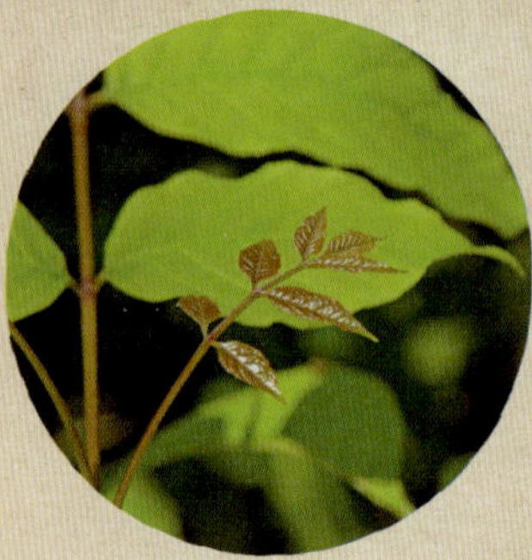

Ash is the tree of order and balance

of Scotland, ash represented the female ancestors of humanity and was known as the loving, all-embracing World Mother. It was seen as the feminine counterpart to the father tree, the mighty oak. Across the ocean, the ash tree maintained similar legends. In Haudenosaunee (Algonquin) lore, it was held that humankind began when the Creator shot an arrow into the heart of an ash tree and humans, both male and female, emerged.

Meeting Ash

As an excellent colonizer, white ash helps form the backbone of northern temperate forests. Along with basswood and black cherry, they are among the first hardwoods to set root, aiding in the reestablishment of deciduous forests, and their dappled shade makes them ideal nurse trees for oaks, maples and hickories.

The straight, opposite branches and thick, rigid twigs are very noticeable from a distance, and the compound leaves are assembled in opposite pairs. White ash is stunning in autumn, showing a distinctive misty, purple-maroon that contrasts well with the bright colours of maples. The fruit are winged seeds, known as samaras or keys, and are shaped like canoe paddles. They remain on the tree throughout the winter months until the wind blows them off. The aerodynamic shape allows them to spin when falling, carrying them a considerable distance from their parents.

Tree of Order and Balance

Ash is regarded as the tree of balance and universal order; the marriage of opposites that link the outer and inner worlds. This symmetry is seen in its physical features, such as its opposite branches and balanced compound-leaf structure. The limbs stretch into the heavens and the roots grow deep into the earth, symbolizing perfect harmony and balance; as above, so below. To those experiencing a polarized existence, this equilibrium offers stability. In a number of cultures, ash is considered to have both male and female energy. Its thick, straight, masculine branch tips reach toward the sky, but the feathery leaves have a graceful, feminine appearance. It is ruled by the male energy of the sun but has a special relationship with the female element of water.

The Tree of Equality

Ash was one of the traditional woods used for Yule logs. Kindling the home fires during the Winter Solstices with Yggdrasil, "the tree of life," symbolized the death of the old year and the beginning of a new. This act was believed to ensure prosperity in the year ahead. As well, burning coppiced ash sticks tightly bound together into faggots was a widespread Yule or Christmastide custom. These bundles are still prepared for use in pubs and domestic hearths, and it is customary that the oldest person in the establishment place them on the fire.

Connected to balance and harmony, ash was also recognized as the tree of equality. When laid on fires during the Feast of Yule, master and servants were then on an equal footing, allowing them to socialize and play games freely through the night. During the burning, fun and merriment commenced, and any bursting of the bonds that tied the faggots signaled all those present to drink up. The refreshments usually consisted of ale, cider, eggnog or hot punch, and a great deal of cheering accompanied each round. Wassailers would walk through villages with their ashen faggots, singing songs with the expectation they would be invited in for drinks. Another related custom was to tie the faggot with three or more bindings, each of these chosen by a young person. The bond first to burst in the fire would indicate who would be first to marry.

Medicinal Uses

The bark and leaves have some limited medicinal uses and are employed in circumstances where a bitter tonic and an astringent are deemed useful. As a diuretic it helps balance the water within the body and is traditionally used to prevent obesity due to water retention. It has proven beneficial in the treatment of urinary tract infections and helps rectify a buildup of metabolic waste. This makes it especially useful for gout and rheumatic complaints, breaking up kidney stones, and treating some forms of rashes. Matthew Wood suggests that its astringent qualities make it beneficial for tissue states that are lax or atrophied. He noted that it has been highly recommended as a remedy for a prolapsed uterus, irregularity of menses and painful periods due to congestion.

The Wood

At one time, ash wood would have been cherished and heavily used in the British Isles. Trees were not only cut for lumber, but, similar to today, forests were cleared for development, leaving scars on the landscape. In 1664, a large castle being built at Portmore (in County Antrim, Northern Ireland) by Lord Conway of England required that the trees that stood in the way be removed. A poem written in the 1700s regarding the trees' "woeful destruction" was put to music and first published in 1840 by Edward Bunting's *Ancient Music of Ireland*. The following verse laments its devastation:

All the birds in the forest, they bitterly weep

Saying, "where will we shelter or where will we sleep?"

For the oak and the ash, they are all cutten down

And the walls of Bonny Portmore are all down to the ground

Ash timber continues to be highly valued for its strength, toughness and elasticity, always fetching a good price. Because it is impressively strong, flexible and shock-resistant, it is the material of choice for such items as baseball bats, hockey sticks, tennis racquets, polo mallets and lacrosse sticks, and many home runs have been hit and goals scored with the help of this tree. Ash forests near Louisville were harvested to make the famed Louisville slugger baseball bats; however, over the years, many athletics have turned to wood that has grown in the northern forests of Pennsylvania, New York and Canada because its slower growth and tighter grain results in a better-quality product. These same assets also made it useful for hay forks, scythes and ladders, and today, handles for axes, hoes and shovels continue to be made of ash. The Anishinaabe (Ojibwe) people employed it for such purposes as sleds, canoe ribs, snowshoe frames and canoe paddles. Even Henry Thoreau reported, "no wood is equal to our ash for oars, so pliant and elastic and strong."

Coppice Growth

In Europe it was common practice to coppice ash. This involved cutting the tree back to the ground every ten years or so and allowing it to regrow new suckers. The natural life span of an ash tree is around 200 years, but a stump from a coppiced tree seems to be able to produce strong, straight poles suitable for fishing spears, oars, walking sticks and fire wood almost indefinitely. An eighteen-foot-diameter coppiced stool in Suffolk has been estimated to be over 1000 years old.

Black Ash Baskets

Along with sugar maple, white birch and white cedar, black ash is a fundamental component of the Indigenous culture. Not only is it a primary resource, it is also an important ceremonial tree contributing to the richness of their traditions. It is commonly known as "basket ash," because it is the material of choice for the famous ash splint baskets made by the Indigenous people of eastern North America. Their techniques of basket making have been passed down through the generations, and their baskets were made for both utilitarian and ceremonial purposes.

Blue Ash Dye

The native blue ash, from which a blue dye is extracted from the inner bark, was employed by the Native Americans as a colouring. The sap turns blue when exposed to air, and a freshly broken twig or piece of bark, when steeped in a glass of water, will turn the liquid blue. The geometric scientific name, *Fraxinus quadrangulata*, was derived from its distinctive square or four-sided twigs.

Wood for Firelight

The dense wood of ash burns for a long time with ample heat and little smoke, making it highly valued for firewood. In fact, so ideal is it for this purpose that the botanical name *Fraxinus* means firelight. The wood contains flammable oils, chemically similar to olive oil, making it easy to light whether seasoned or in a fresh, green state. Walter de la Mare wrote in his poem *Trees*, "*Of all the trees in England, Her sweet three corners in, only the Ash, the bonnie Ash, burns fierce while it is green.*" Ash brought light into the hearth at Winter Solstice, and in Ireland, ash twigs were used to "lighten-up" slow-smoldering peat fires. This practice was adopted by the early pioneers in Canada, using ash to start their cook stoves. A poem depicting the quality of different fuel wood states the value of ash.

Beech wood fires are
bright and clear,
If the logs are kept a year;
Chestnut's only good, they say,
If for long, it's laid away;
Make a fire of elder tree,
Death within your house shall be;
But ash new or ash old,
Is fit for a queen with
a crown of gold

Birch and fir logs burn too fast,
Blaze up bright and do not last;
It is by the Irish said,
Hawthorn bakes the sweetest bread;
Elm wood (English elm)
burns like churchyard mold,
E'en the very flames are cold;
But ash green or ash brown,
Is fit for a queen with
a golden crown

Poplar gives a bitter smoke,
Fills your eyes and
makes you choke;
Applewood will scent your room,
With an incense-like perfume;
Oaken logs if dry and old,
Keep away the winter's cold;
But ash wet or ash dry,
A king shall warm his slippers by
~Anonymous~

Protective Qualities

In the *Language of Flowers*, ash symbolizes grandeur. To the ancient Irish, the ash tree held great magical importance and was one of the three guardian trees that protected their land. So powerful, that in the sixteenth century, merely carrying the winged keys shielded one from the malicious influences of sorcerers. Sticks of ash were used to drive cattle, as it was believed they were gifted with qualities that ensured no harm would come to them. Even today, ash leaves and twigs are placed in cars to provide protection against any mishaps or accidents.

Wood for Spears, Staffs, Wands and Broomsticks

In early Celtic traditions, ash was considered the best wood for spears, staffs, walking sticks and arrow shafts in the belief it had great magical powers. In fact, the name *ash* may have been derived from the Anglo-Saxon word *asec*, a term used for a ritualistic spear. In many cultures, the staff became, in essence, a portable version of the World Tree, connecting the user to the realms of earth and sky. The Druids carried magical ash staffs to safeguard themselves while traveling and placed them by entrance ways before entering buildings to ensure defense against harmful influences.

The jostling stick with which Little John bested Robin Hood was most certainly crafted of ash, and in *The Lord of the Rings*, the Wizard Gandalf is said to have carried an ash staff. The practice of fighting with staffs was known as staving, an expression that has survived to present day. To use the term "staving off disasters" we refer to the age when ash staffs were used to fight fierce battles. Interestingly, despite its use in weaponry, ash was also seen as having an influence in "checking the powers of peace" and was believed to bring harmony to a situation by resolving conflicts.

In archaeological digs in Wales, wands carved from ash dating from the early part of the first century were found, evidence that this wood was revered and employed by the ancient Druids. These ash wands were believed to have been used to raise and direct healing energy and carry out enchantments.

The traditional witch's broomstick or besom was constructed of three different woods, each providing different magical benefits. The handle was made of ash, while birch twigs, which formed the brush, were tied with willow bindings. The ash wood represented protection and strength, birch drew spirits to one's service and willow connected them to the goddess energy.

A Charm against Snakes

Likely accounting for its protective qualities, there are many literary references describing ash's charm-like powers against venomous snakes. According to folklore, no poison could exist within the shadow of an ash, and snakes in particular have an innate fear of them. John Gerard, English botanist and herbalist of the sixteenth century, wrote, "The leaves of this tree are of so great a virtue against serpents as that they dare not so much as touch the morning and evening shadow of the tree, but shun them afar off." Even in North America, people were convinced that ash leaves, when stuffed in moccasins or boots, were highly offensive to serpents and would prevent them from biting. One French missionary in Quebec claimed "one never finds serpents in the swamps where this tree abounds." He went on to say, "Where Canadians think there are serpents and venomous beasts, they only have to strew the leaves or branches and immediately not a live one among them is left ... it is an undoubted fact that these vipers flee the scent of ash."

In Ireland, ash cradles were believed to shield babies from snakes, and Saint Patrick was said to have driven the serpents out of Ireland with the aid of an ash stick. Curiously, in ancient Celtic mythology, serpents are a symbol of wisdom, rebirth and a connection to the female aspect of earth energy. There is some speculation then that when St. Patrick was eradicating the snakes in Ireland, he may have actually been trying to suppress the power women held or reject the ancient wisdom of the culture.

Water Protection

Ash represents March in the Celtic tree calendar, the month of the floods. It has a special affinity with water and represents the power that resides within it. Because of this relationship, ash trees, along with hawthorns, were often planted beside Irish holy wells and springs to protect the purity of the water. On the Isle of Man, old ash stumps have been found near these sacred wells, suggesting its association with healing and granting wishes.

Considered a superior guardian tree, it was carried on long journeys for protection and guidance. For those going to sea, small, equal-armed solar crosses carved of ash wood were carried on boats to ensure sailors a safe voyage and protection from drowning.

Tree of Healing

Ash was reputed for its ability to cure ailing children, especially those suffering from physical disorders such as ruptures, hernias or weak limbs. In order to start the healing process and charm away the issue, the child was passed through a cleft in an ash sapling at sunrise. When young and flexible, the sapling was split lengthwise down the trunk and wedges were inserted to create an opening sufficient enough to accommodate the child without touching either side of the tree. After the ceremony, the tree was carefully bound up, and as it grew together, the patient's health would improve and outgrow any infirmities. Hereafter, there was an intimate bond between the tree and patient and it was imperative that it not be cut or harmed during the individual's lifetime. The state of the tree reflected the person's health and strength, leading people to become, understandably, somewhat protective of "their" ash tree. Even today this formality still prevails in parts of rural England and caretakers of arboretums tell of cases where babies are brought to ancient ash trees on the grounds that in the past have proven healing qualities.

At one time, newborns in the British Isles were given a teaspoon of ash sap, believing this would prevent disease and infant mortality. At the birthing, the midwife would place one end of a green ash stick in the fire. While it was burning, the sap would ooze out of the other end of the stick which would be collected on a spoon.

A Tree for Luck and Love

The compound leaf of an ash usually holds an odd number of leaflets, and to find one with an even number, or one without a terminal leaflet, was considered as lucky as finding a four-leaf clover. Picking such a leaf was believed to bring positive energy, prosperity and personal fortune especially if the following verse was spoken:

Even ash, I do thee pluck
Hoping this to meet good luck
If no luck I get from thee
I shall wish thee on the tree

This same "even ash leaf" was also used in love divinations. In Northern England, it was said that if a maiden placed such leaves under her pillow, she would have prophetic dreams of her future husband. As well, if she wished to determine her forthcoming love, she could pick an "even ash leaf" and say:

Even ash, even ash, I
pluck thee off the tree,
The first man I meet, my
true love he shall be

If she then placed the leaf in her left shoe, soon after, he most certainly would make his appearance.

Predicting the Weather

Weather was often forecasted from natural signs, and of course trees were the source of many predictions. Like oak, it seemed that ash attracted lightning, hence the expression "avoid the ash, for it courts the flash," and it was well advised not to stand under this tree during an electrical storm. Ash was considered one of the chosen trees of Thor, the god of thunder and lightning, because it was able to remain alive even after the celestial fires descended on it. Because it bore the brunt of many lightning strikes, the ancient Greeks used ash in rituals to encourage rain.

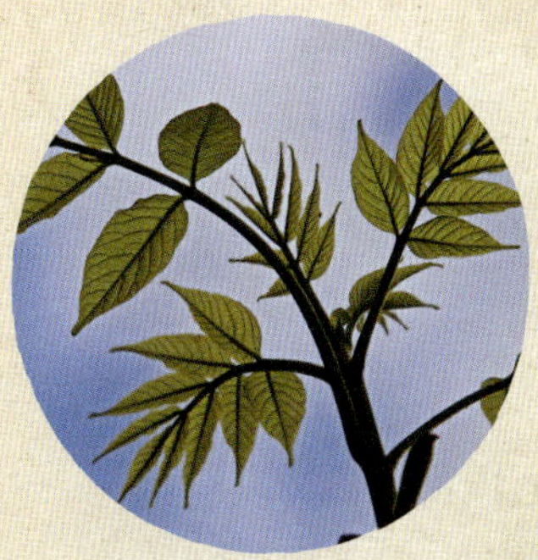

Ash and oak were used to predict the amount of rainfall in the upcoming season

Ash and oak could also determine how wet the upcoming season would be, as depicted in this verse:

If the oak is out before the ash
We shall only have a splash
If the ash is out before the oak
We shall surely have a soak

Meaning, if the ash tree produces leaves before the oak, the summer will be wet.

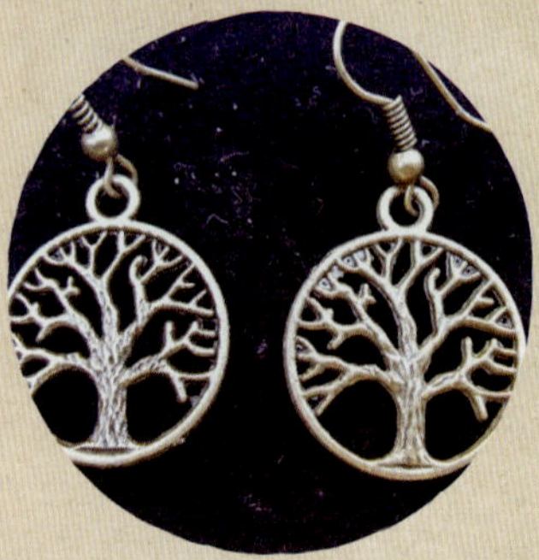

The "Great World Tree" or "Tree of Life" is often depicted on jewelry

It goes on to say:

If oak and ash leaves show together
Us may fear some awful weather
This be a sight but seldom seen
That could remind
us what has been

Folklore

After thorn, ash and oak are the most commonly used tree in the naming of places, towns and villages in the English countryside.

In early England, it was believed that if ash trees failed to produce seed, disaster was foretold and future ventures would be unsuccessful. This barrenness was a sure sign of public calamity and predicted the death of a member of the royal family. Therefore, the king would give a great deal of money to someone who could produce a branch with keys during sparse years.

There doesn't appear to be any apparent reason why this tree is connected with Ash Wednesday except for the obvious association with the word. However, in parts of England, ash twigs were carried to school on Ash Wednesday by children. Anyone who failed to produce a twig when asked ran the risk of having their feet stomped on by others who possessed one. This custom ended at midday, and the twigs were disposed of by noon.

Ash had a reputation for magically curing warts. When a wart was rubbed on the bark, it was thought to be absorbed into the tree if these words were spoken;

Ashen tree, ashen tree
May you take these warts off me

Burying a newborn's first nail clippings beneath an ash ensured the child would grow up to be a good singer.

Ash, oak and hawthorn make up the triad of powerful fairy trees, and these trees should never be harmed. If you want to increase your chances of seeing fairies, look where all three grow together.

Lessons of Ash

Ash can heal the loneliness of the human spirit that is out of touch with its origins and feels removed from nature and the cycle of the year. The natural forces on Earth are linked to the "Great World Ash"; therefore, this tree promotes a feeling of being "in tune" with our surroundings and provides us a deep sense of purpose and belonging.

Through a continual progression of balance and marrying opposites, ash can help bring these attributes into our life and achieve harmony within. It encourages us to gain strength and competence so that we might better understand ourselves. As in the ancient Druid practice, carrying ash is a way to draw upon your own power, build knowledge and skills and develop self-mastery. It also aids in communication, intelligence and wisdom and promotes curiosity. It removes mental blockages and acts as a poetic muse to inspire writers, poets and scholars.

White Birch

Betula papyrifera

Silver Birch, Paper Birch, Canoe Birch, Canoe Tree, Moon Birch, Moon Mother, Silver Maiden, White Goddess, Lady of the Woods and Ribbon Tree

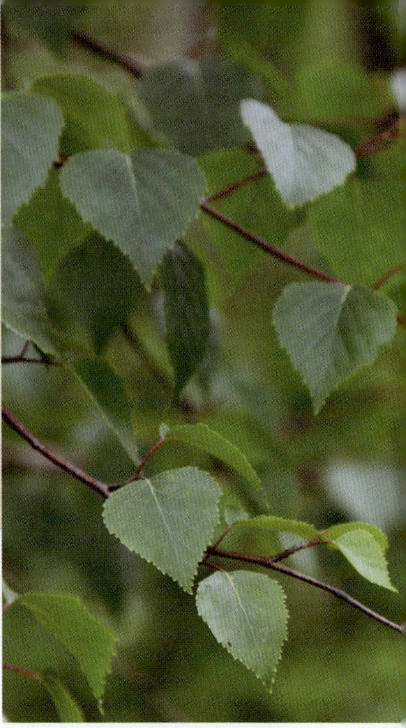

Of all the trees, birch is considered one of the most graceful. Its beauty is observed as its delicate, slender branches sway and dance in the breeze like some eloquent choreography, and its flowing femininity easily evokes images of young women dancing in the moonlight. It is associated with the element air, and as the wind moves through its foliage, the fluttering leaves gently whisper messages to those who dwell in the forest. Revered by many northern cultures, it is one of the most poetic trees and for centuries has been depicted in poetry, art, songs and fairy tales.

The Lady of the Woods

Each tree has its own energy or expression, and the birch releases an agile, flowing pattern. Because of her feminine presence, poet S.T. Coleridge called her the "Lady of the Woods," lending beauty without grandeur. Although its fragile features reveal a gentle quality, there is nothing feeble about this tree. It is one of the most resilient species, being able to take hold in inhospitable environments where others are unable to grow. As a pioneer species, birch, along with poplar, has a remarkable aptitude for being the first to set root in clear-cut areas or after fires, marking the early transitional phase in the creation of a forest. Considered the oldest tree of the north, this ancient plant was one of the initial trees to colonize poor, thin soils after the last ice age, when the ice caps retreated 13,000 years ago. It thrives in high altitudes and cold climates, making it well suited to unseasonable northern woods, and the supple branches are very sturdy in storms, capable of bending in heavy snow and ice.

Birch provides an important service to forest ecosystems. As a fast-growing, short-lived nurse tree, it casts light shade and offers shelter to slower growing species. It lives just long enough for the next generation of trees, such as ash, basswood and oaks, to take root and is eventually shaded out by these more shade-tolerant species. Like a mother figure, not only does she prepare the way and provide protection for slower growing saplings but the leaves and wood also decay readily, bringing fertility to the earth and improving the environment for others within the community.

Meeting Birch

Birch is relatively short-lived, seldom existing more than 80 years, but what it lacks in grand stature or impressive age it makes up in sheer beauty. It is a popular tree in the horticultural trade, being a valued specimen in small gardens for every season. It is one of the first trees to burst into leaf in spring, and in autumn the bright yellow foliage puts on a spectacular show. The young stems are a warm reddish-brown colour, and the trunk doesn't develop its silvery bark for the first decade. It then provides a stunning impact in the landscape on clear nights when the snowy, white trunks shine in the moonlight. When planted along garden paths, it also makes a nice addition in sensory gardens, where the exfoliating bark can be explored.

The bark peels off in strips, making it easily recognized even by children. The reflective, white bark protects this pioneer tree from sun scald while inhabiting open environments. This is a cold-climate adaptation that prevents the bark from heating on sunny winter days, causing the trunk to crack.

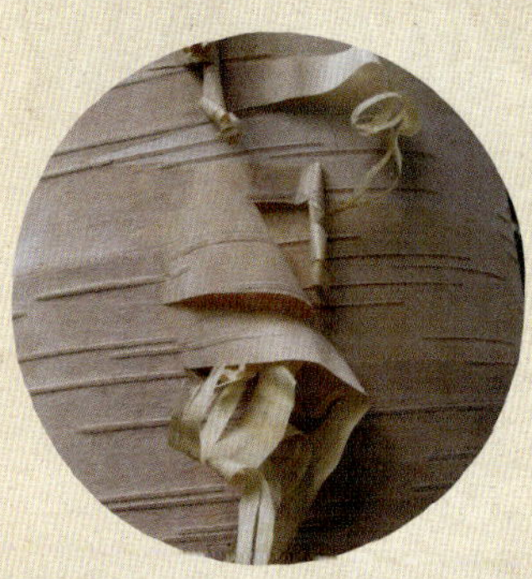

The stunning white bark

Although the wood itself rots readily, its bark is very durable and water resistant. When a tree dies, this outer skin is the last to decay and remains intact long after the inner wood has decomposed. If

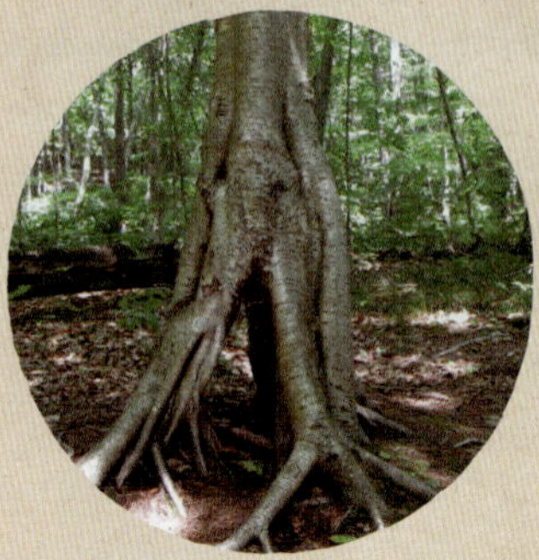

The stilted roots of yellow birch

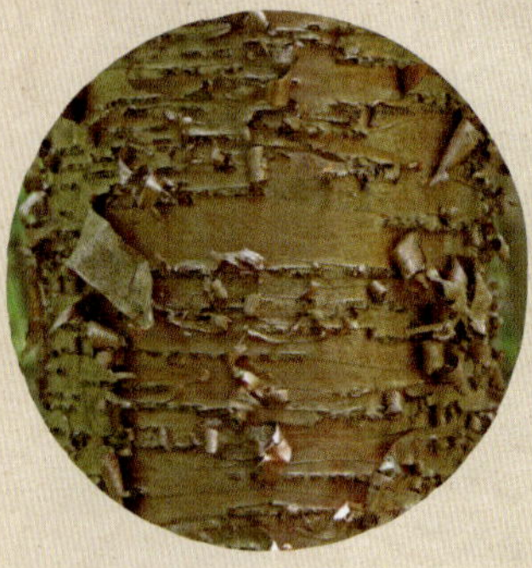

The lustrous, golden bark of yellow birch

you climb upon a fallen log that appears solid, you may be surprised to find yourself stepping right through the hollow shell.

A close cousin, yellow birch (*Betula alleghaniensis*), has unique lustrous, golden bark that peels in small ragged curls. The twigs, when crushed or scratched, reveal their delightfully fragrant oils, which are similar to that of wintergreen (*Gaultheria procumbens*). This biochemical, also found in black birch (*Betula lenta*), affords both odour and flavour and is known as methyl salicylate. It was once considered important medicine to help reduce fevers, ease pain and decrease inflammation.

Seed Germination

White birch likes its fair share of sunlight and will not tolerate shade. It is often found in pure stands, forming beautiful, airy groves, or in even-aged stands with fir, spruce and cedar. The seeds are not able to sprout on leaf litter, but instead need bare soil with plenty of light in order to germinate. On the other hand, yellow birch is more shade-tolerant and is rarely found in pure stands. It enjoys rich, moist soils and grows with white pine, hemlock, beech, and sugar maple. Here too, leaf litter impedes seed germination; however, yellow birch is well adapted to sprouting on rotting stumps and logs. This is easily observed when walking through moist forests. Once germinated, the roots grow around the stump or log, and after these structures decay the tree is frequently left perched on stilted roots.

Insect and Spider Relationships

A wealth of insect species can be observed feeding on birch. Several butterfly and moth caterpillars use it as a host plant, including the white admiral and tiger swallowtail. Birch also has a unique relationship with spiders. Orb spiders spin a new web daily, and many consume the old one to recycle the silk protein and recover some energy spent in web making. In the spring, birch produces abundant airborne pollen, which becomes caught in these silky structures. Thus, the spiders inevitably dine on the ensnared pollen, which is highly nutritious for both the spiders and their young.

Wildlife Value

Tree species with exfoliating bark, such as birch, provides lots of nooks and crannies where insects conceal themselves during the winter months. In turn, these insects supply food for chickadees, nuthatches and woodpeckers at a time of year when food is limited. Birch also supplies many more benefits to wildlife. The seeds remain in the catkins through the winter, contributing important nourishment for resident song birds such as red polls, pine siskins and chickadees, and the leaf buds are consumed by large game birds, including grouse and wild turkey. When available, vireos and black throated green warblers use the peeling bark strips for constructing their nest. Mammals, such as deer, rabbits and hares, enjoy browsing on the twigs, particularly that of yellow birch.

Holes drilled in regular horizontal lines around the trunk, resembling a necklace, are an indication that yellow bellied sapsuckers have been feeding. Although not the only tree they tap, birch is one of their favorites. After creating the holes, they return periodically to consume the oozing sap and investigative insects. Secondary feeders, such as ruby throated hummingbirds and downy woodpeckers, are also attracted to the sweet liquid.

Commonly found on the trunks of birch and aspen is a tough, hoof-shaped fungus, known as the horseshoe or false tinder fungus (*Fomes fomentarius*), and its presence is an indication of heartwood rot. This disease causes more loss of timber than any other hardwood fungus, and when a tree is infected, the wood rots quickly. Affected trees provide potential cavity trees for nesting birds as well as foraging sites for woodpeckers that are attracted to the large array of insects living in the rotting wood. Another fungus association is the beautiful fly agaric toadstool, which forms a symbiotic relationship with birch and is often found growing among them. This hallucinogenic mushroom has a scarlet red cap with white dots and is included in all good fairy tales.

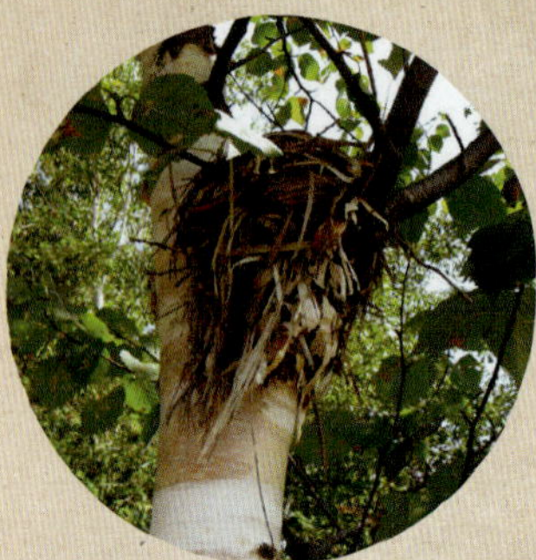

Red-eyed vireo nest made of white birch bark

Meaning of its Name

The linguistic root of *birch* is unclear. The name is thought to be derived from the Sanskrit word *bhurga*, which literally means a "tree whose bark is used to write upon." However, some claim it came from *bhura*, signifying "bright" or "shining" tree, no doubt in reference to the beautiful white bark; while others believe it may be from the Anglo-Saxon word *beorgan*, meaning "to protect" or "shelter."

The specific name for white birch is *papyrifera*, which implies paper-bearing, and again references the distinctive creamy, white bark that peels away from the trunk like paper. The bark is also the basis for many of its common names, including paper birch, silver birch, canoe birch, moon birch, moon mother, silver maiden and white goddess.

Birch Sap

Before leaf emergence, birch can be tapped in spring as a source of sap. This produces a clear, refreshing beverage straight from the tree, and the ancient Druids made it into cordial to celebrate the Spring Equinox. Similar to maples, the sap can be simmered down into golden brown syrup. Birch produces its spring flow slightly later than maple; therefore, the spigots and buckets from the recently shut down maple trees can be transferred over to the birch. However, the season is shorter and birch sap is half as sweet as maple, taking approximately 80 to 100 litres of sap to make 1 litre of syrup.

In many northern cultures, the slightly sweet sap was fermented into delicious birch wine, healthy beer, and mead, and this process is still practiced in the Scottish Highlands to recognize the coming of spring. In America, another domestic drink was birch beer. This was made from a twig and inner bark infusion of the yellow and black birch and carbonated water to create a drink similar to commercial root beer. Its flavouring and odour are produced by the "wintergreen" essential oils contained within the tree.

Culinary Uses

The twigs and inner bark also create a delightful tea, and the young leaves and catkins make a nice addition to salads. The inner bark is high in protein and naturally sweet, rendering it a nutritious emergency famine food. This alternative food source may have saved hundreds of Confederate soldiers in 1861 during their retreat in Virginia, and for years after, their route could be traced by the peeled birch trees. They added it to soups and stews, or dried and ground it into meal and combined it with other flours to make breads and ash cakes.

Medicinal Uses

Although more widely known for their utilitarian benefits, various birch species have also been used in northern cultures for their healing virtues. Like tree sap stirring in early spring, birch gets the energy flowing. There are several important healing constituents in white birch, but it is mainly the betulin within the plant that converts to betulinic acid in the body that provides its medicinal assets. Betulin is seen in the snowy white pigment in the bark, which comes off on your fingers when gently rubbed. The fresh leaves and inner bark also make a mild, astringent tea or topical oil.

Benefitting the Kidneys

The leaves, twigs and inner bark of white birch bring healing energy to the kidneys. A tea drunk in spring is an excellent cleansing tonic and detoxifier that helps clear sluggishness and congestion. It mainly works through the urinary tract as a non-irritating diuretic to remove waste products without overworking the system. As well, by influencing the kidneys, it has a reputation for reducing fluid retention, such as cardiac or renal edema, and due to its mild, antiseptic qualities, it effectively clears cystitis and other urinary tract infections. Furthermore, it is a reliable solvent for preventing and eliminating gravel and breaking up kidney and bladder stones. Like dandelion, it is rich in potassium and does not deplete the body of this important mineral the way other medical diuretics do.

Joints and Muscles

The supple branches seem to indicate its aptitude for resolving rheumatic conditions, arthritic deposits and gout. This cleansing diuretic has the ability to remove waste products from the blood and is an excellent remedy for musculoskeletal issues due to a buildup of toxins in the joints. The inner bark or infused leaf oil can also be applied externally to ease muscle aches and pains.

Additionally, the leaves and twigs of yellow and black birch are a good source of methyl salicylate or wintergreen oil, rendering them a helpful analgesic. Birch oil is used topically for its fast-acting anti-inflammatory and aspirin-like properties to ease arthritic pain, rheumatic complaints, fibromyalgia, aching joints, neuralgia, painful tendons, stiff muscles and strains.

Skin Issues

Within its natural range, white birch has had a longstanding tradition for aiding with skin complaints, and according to the Doctrine of Signatures this is indicated by the bark's resemblance to the skin. Its skin healing qualities are found through a variety of assets. First, it is an excellent cleansing tonic and diuretic, assisting the lymphatics and supporting the kidneys to clear sluggishness and remove waste products. An accumulation of toxins in the body often shows itself as skin issues. Secondly, it is considered a mild diaphoretic, which helps open the sweat glands, thereby detoxifying the system through perspiration. Lastly, birch's astringent, antiseptic and anti-inflammatory properties all contribute to skin healing.

A strong tea made from the leaves or twigs effectively aids healing and has a reputation for treating many severe skin ailments and eruptions, such as eczema, psoriasis, rashes, acne, skin lesions, ulcers, boils, cuts, wounds and burns. It reliably removes dry, hardened, mineralized skin and rarely fails when used on poison ivy. Whenever possible, it is best to help the remedial process by employing birch both internally and externally.

Chaga Mushroom

There is another gift of the northern woods that grows on birch trees known as the chaga mushroom (*Inonotus obliquus*) or clinker polypore. Chaga is slow-growing and long-lived, preferring cold forests throughout the northern hemisphere. It looks like a clump of blackened cinder or a crusty formation resembling a bursting tumor rather than a mushroom.

Betulin, which is naturally present in birch bark, is converted into betulinic acid by the mushroom, making it readily available within the body. Betulinic acid has recently attracted interest in the fight against cancer because it has been found to directly target and destroy cancer cells and has demonstrated strong anti-tumor activities. Chaga is also recognized as a powerful immunomodulator, helping to boost the immune system. To further its reputation as a medicinal mushroom, it has adaptogen qualities that help bring the body back into balance; has beneficial effects on the nervous system to reduce stress; and exhibits antioxidant properties that mitigate the damaging effects of free radicals.

Cosmetic Uses

The astringent sap has a gentle action on the complexion and in the past was commonly used by those with sensitive skin. Birch has a long history as a hair tonic, and both a rinse and oil were rubbed on the scalp to encourage hair growth or improve scalp health. Yellow birch twigs were chewed, and the softened ends were used much like a toothbrush for oral hygiene.

Birch Wood

White Birch has an unusual trait of showing no difference between the inner heartwood and sapwood. Because of its rapid life cycle, it produces weak, soft timber; however, even though the wood is not particularly hard wearing or durable, for thousands of years it was the mainstay of human settlement in the cold north, where little else grew. Here it was employed for all manner of household gadgets, agricultural implements and general building material, and was used to make everything from houses to furniture, dishes, ploughs and carts. Historically, it was in great demand for reels and bobbins in the cotton industry, and birch continues to be used for humble purposes, such as spools for thread, clothespins, dowels, buckets, broom handles, wooden toys and pulp for the manufacturing of paper.

On the other hand, yellow birch wood is hard and dense, and some woodworkers compare it to maple. Early colonists used it for ox yokes, and during World War II it formed airplane frames. Today it is used for making furniture, flooring, plywood and high-quality veneer, and its straight grain makes it suitable for turning. While harvesting, some trees may show a curly grain, which is prized for cabinets and is often marketed as "Canadian silky wood."

The oils saturated in the bark and wood fibers are highly combustible and burn well even when the wood is green, thus making useful kindling. Though it produces a sweet smell while burning, an old poem that depicts the quality of fuel wood stated that "birch logs burn too fast, blaze up bright and do not last." Despite this, in the Scottish Highlands birch was employed as fuel for smoking ham and herring.

Using the Bark

Because the thin bark is durable and peels readily, the Indigenous people made it into any number of items. Heat from fire made it incredibly pliable, and it was easily stretched into any form required. The trees were only chopped on one side so that when they fell, they would rest on the stump instead of the ground, thereby preventing the bark from becoming soiled.

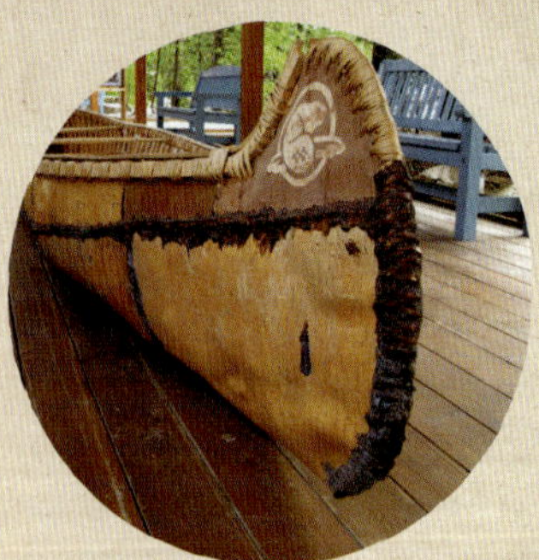

A traditional birch bark canoe

Birch Bark Canoes

White birch is most famous for making bark canoes, and from this use it became known as "canoe birch." The Ojibway (Anishinaabe) people made canoe building an exquisite art. Their creations were strong, durable and flexible, and owing to their light weight they were easily lifted onto the shoulders and carried over land so that the people could freely travel all over the country. Turned upside down, they doubled as a shelter in inclement weather. These crafts were very sturdy, able to shoot rapids and brave oceans, and the French voyageurs, quickly adopted them to cross 3000 miles of Canadian waters to establish fur trading routes in the far northwest. They survived most disasters, lasting up to ten years, but if damage occurred, they could easily be repaired at any time with material found in the forest.

Lacking available birch, canoes were also made with other types of bark, with elm, hickory and basswood being common substitutes. A common failing was that these shells absorbed water, becoming waterlogged and heavy, and were less efficient than the light, waterproof birch bark canoes.

Shelters, Dishes and Storage Containers

The light bark was employed for teepees and to waterproof shelters, being used in much the same way that roofing paper is used today. Moreover, it was fashioned into bark cups, plates and bowls for drinking and eating, and made into cooking kettles. These vessels could be filled with water and placed on the fire. The bark above the water level might burn, but the section below the liquid would last long enough to cook meat or boil water for tea. Birch bark baskets or containers, known as *makuks*, were also made to hold food items such as beans, corn, peas, maple sugar, dried meat and fish. Due to the bark's antifungal properties, food or preserves stored in birch containers would last longer and circumvent decay and mold.

Paper, Tinder, and Torches

The bark separates into thin layers, and its use as water-resistant writing paper goes back to ancient times. It was employed as a replacement for oiled paper for writing journals, particularly by early voyageurs. It was favoured over other paper because it lasted longer, due to the fact it didn't readily absorb moisture or go moldy.

The bark is also a camper's best friend. It is highly flammable and a reliable fire starter even in the wettest weather, and it is said that "no day is so damp that this bark won't flare into a blaze." As well, the Indigenous people rolled the bark into cylinders to form torches, which could be stuck upright in the ground around their camp in the evenings.

Russian Leather

Oils extracted from birch bark continue to be used in the tanning process in Russia, especially where large birch forests exist. Russian leather differs from other types of leather because, after the tanning process is complete, birch oil is worked into the product. This final stage of curing the hide gives the leather durability and flexibility and imparts water resistance. As well, due to birch oil's fungicidal qualities, Russian leather has historically been used to bind books because it is less liable to become moldy or incur insect damage. The oil is still used on stored saddles, harness and bridles that are prone to mildew.

Brooms and Besoms

Birch has a long tradition in broom making. Such brooms usually resemble a large whisk or the sort of broom ridden by witches at Halloween. Indeed, the traditional brooms of witches, known as besoms, were allegedly made from bundles of birch twigs that were bound and tied with willow around an ash handle. These birch brooms were used to drive out the old year on the morning after the Winter Solstice (Yule), or at Samhain (Halloween), the start of the Celtic year. A new year could not start until the old one had finished and all harmful influences were cast away; therefore, they metaphorically swept out old or malign spirits from the hearth. These brooms were also used in a ritual known as "beating the bounds." Here the boundaries of the property were walked and marked with the besom to rid the area of evil spirits, provide protective qualities and increase fertility by requesting the spirits of the land to ensure a bountiful harvest. In the same way, birch brooms were used to purify gardens.

On a practical note, birch brooms are still made for their unique ability to lift damp leaves from the lawn. They are favoured for sweeping cobblestone patios and brushing fresh snow from paths, and the Scottish used them to sweep the ice during curling games. The Irish besom wedding was considered legal even into the nineteenth century (some Irish still regards it so). During the ceremony, a besom of birch is held at the doorway of their home, and when the couple jumps over it, they are wed.

New Beginnings and Renewed Life

Birch is the tree of new beginnings, renewed life, springtime and purification. As a pioneer species, it is one of the first trees to recolonize a disturbed area and quick to leaf out in spring. It is only fitting then that birch symbolizes the first moon in the Celtic calendar and the first letter of Ogham, the Celtic tree alphabet. Yule logs were traditionally made of birch and it was customary to burn them in midwinter fires to drive out the spirit of the old year while welcoming in the new. This practice connected the inhabitants with a fresh start, new hope and the promise of what was to come. Christians continued this tradition by burning birch logs for each day of the twelve days of Christmas to celebrate the birth of Christ. Likewise, the young, supple branches were used to decorate churches at the beginning of Pentecost or Whit Sunday (Whitsuntide) to denote a new start and rebirth after the Easter season. This tradition is still maintained in some areas of Great Britain. Possibly due to its bright white bark, birch is also considered a powerful light bringer and was used at Imbolc festivals (February 2) or Candlemas to encourage the returning light and rebirth of the sun.

Symbol of Fertility and Love

Birch has a strong fertility connection and was also associated with Beltane festivities (May 1), where spring, love and fruitfulness were celebrated and young couples frolicked in birch groves. Birch logs were burned in Beltane fires, thus encouraging the renewal of fertile vigor to the awakening Earth. May poles of birch were decorated with colourful ribbons and shiny objects, becoming the focal point of villages. Old fertility dances were performed around the poles with much singing and drinking, while wrapping them with ribbon to ensure health and abundant crops. These "ribbon trees," as they were sometimes known, are still popular in many rural areas of Ireland. Ribbons also adorned trunks of living birches so no harm came to the tree.

Birch is an obvious choice in fertility rites to represent the emergence of spring, new awakenings and life-giving forces. Tossing a birch twig into a stream was a charm to bring soft spring rains to fields. It brought blessings to women, for merely touching birch twigs bestowed luck and fertility, and they were given to newlyweds to ensure many children. In the Scottish Highlands, it is rumoured that a barren cow herded with a birch stick would become fertile or a pregnant cow would bear a healthy calf. As a symbol of promised or new love, young maidens in Wales would give their sweetheart a piece of birch as a token of encouragement, indicating that he may begin his courtship.

Symbol of Birth and Mothers

Because birch nurtures new life and symbolizes birth, fresh beginnings and inception, the wood was often used to make baby cradles. These cradles were thought to provide protection to the sleeping child, particularly of a psychic nature, and to prevent kidnapping by fairies. Birch is also seen as the embodiment of feminine energy, providing fertility, grace, nurturing and maternal protectiveness, and it became known as the "mothering tree." It was chosen as the "Mother's Tree" by the American Forestry Association in the 1920s, and sons and daughters were encouraged to plant a birch on Mother's Day in her honour and to deepen their relationship with their mother. This graceful, ladylike tree was planted on the White House grounds for mothers of presidents and in war cemeteries for mothers of soldiers. When addressing the moon phases and the triple goddess (maiden, mother and crone), white birch was associated with the maiden and the waxing phase of the moon.

Folklore

The Celtic people believed that trees carried ancient lessons, and along with oak and yew, birch was one of the three pillars of wisdom. Many rituals were performed within birch groves because of her powerful yet gentle nature. It is also rumoured that fairies and nature spirits inhabit birch circles, and their magic can be drawn upon in times of need.

The peeling bark has long been used as a charm of intent and could rid negative thoughts or those things that were no longer necessary in your life, yet still being held onto. This ritual can be carried out to initiate a change or new beginning, or to cast aside unproductive thoughts. It is particularly effective at New Year's Eve or Halloween, as one-year ends and a new begins. On a piece of birch bark, write down something you want to release from your life and place it on the fire to help rid yourself of this unhelpful influence.

Lessons of Birch

Although she appears fragile, birch is in fact extremely hardy and her strength is unwavering. She has a pioneering spirit that enables her to break new ground and survive under extreme circumstances. Thus, she symbolizes a fresh start and brings courage and determination when taking a new path or starting a new journey. By encouraging new direction and goals, she helps you to envision creative possibilities and can be a source of great strength when coping with potential changes or overcoming difficulties.

Her nurturing properties of offering shelter and protection to others help us with lessons of unselfishness, tolerance and caring for those in need. Moreover, her feminine energies bring grace and elegance into our lives so that we can learn to dance. Her healing spirit reminds us that life is not always a struggle but can be harmonious and sweet. By letting go of our burdens, she allows us to accept the gifts that life has to offer and creates a space for stillness and peace.

White Cedar

Thuja occidentalis

Eastern White Cedar, Arborvitae, Swamp Cedar, Northern White Cedar, Canoe Cedar, Yellow Cedar and Tree of Life

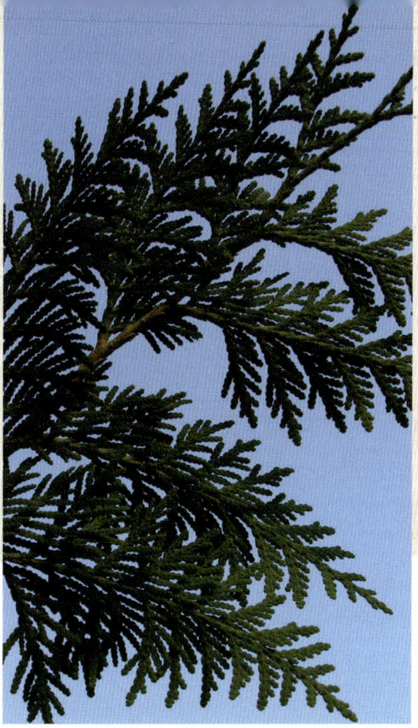

Sometimes referring to her as "Grandmother Tree," the Indigenous people in eastern Canada consider white cedar to be sacred. It was maintained that this revered tree not only housed very powerful spirits that protected the people from harm, it also held the spirits of their departed ancestors. To this day, a special ceremony is procured when felling a cedar, where expressions of gratitude to the tree's spirit are given.

Meeting White Cedar

White cedar is native to central and eastern North America but is often introduced to other regions throughout the world under the name *arborvitae*. Despite its title, this tree is not a true cedar but rather a cypress (*Cupressaceae*) and is not in the same family as the famed cedars of Lebanon (*Cedrus libani*). It naturally grows on two widely differing habitats, seemingly occupying the leftover sites, where it endures little competition from other species. It is found in cold, alkaline swamps and along lake shores and stream borders, but also adapts to windy, exposed conditions on dry, rocky, limestone cliffs and calcareous upland soils. It appears that soil pH is more important for growth than the amount of moisture. Its presence indicates an alkaline environment; therefore, an acidic peat bog will not support white cedar.

In 1840, Canadian naturalist P.H. Gosse wrote "[Cedar] chiefly grows in marshes so densely as to render them almost impenetrable." Seldom occurring as a single specimen, cedar usually prefers

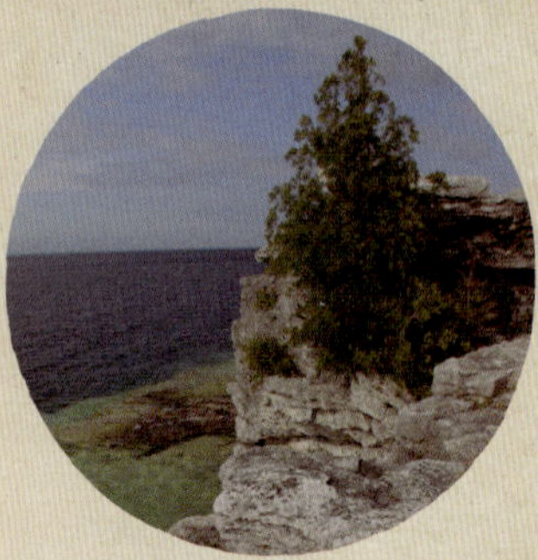

Old cedars on the cliffs of Bruce Peninsula

its own company to that of other trees. They occur in more or less pure stands forming very dense family groupings where light filtering through them generates remarkable beauty. Despite its relatively small stature, cedars are incredibly long-lived trees. Typically, they reach ages of 250 to 300 years, but scientists have found much older specimens on cliff faces overlooking the Great Lakes. Currently the oldest living eastern white cedar is found in Ontario on the Bruce Peninsula. It is over 1000 years old and believed to have germinated around 950. Dead specimens preserved at the bottom of Lake Huron are estimated to be over 1890 years old, the oldest trees in Canada. It is incredible to consider the amount of history these trees may have seen through the years.

Characteristics

Identifying white cedar is relatively easy. The aromatic, flat branches covered with tiny overlapping leaves are quite distinct, and few trees possess soft, evergreen fronds with such intricate patterns. The beautiful reddish trunk, which may show twisting as it ages, is wide at the bottom and decidedly tapered at the growing tip. It is covered in fibrous, stringy bark that is susceptible to fire, making fatalities during forest fires common. As well, due to their shallow root systems, they are vulnerable to wind throw. The large amounts of tannins leached from decaying cedar logs are, in part, the cause of our Northern Ontario lakes and rivers turning a brownish tea-like colour.

On the flat, scale-like leaves there are tiny resin glands, which are the source of cedar's aroma. Each gland holds a small drop of essential oil that when disturbed or warmed by the sun releases a strong, pleasant odour. When walking in cedars, this pungent smell is healing to the spirit and both relaxing and uplifting to the heart.

In the Garden

Cedar is a common tree in the landscape trade, and numerous cultivars of different sizes, colours and growth habits have been developed. In winter, they give life to the landscape, and on warm summer days their aromatic fragrance can be enjoyed along garden paths. As well, they are commonly seen in the rural countryside, acting as shelterbelts to slow wind and protect agricultural fields, water courses and farm buildings.

Cedars also have the ability to absorb solar energy from the sun and trap its heat within their thick foliage. Some of this heat is radiated back into the surrounding environment. This helps produce a microclimate in the garden, thereby increasing planting possibilities and expanding the growing season by warming the beds in early spring and late into the fall.

Meaning of its Name

Members of the cypress family are famous for their essential oils, and all are aromatic. The name *Thuja* is derived from this characteristic. It comes from the Greek word meaning *to fumigate* and the fragrant wood and boughs have long been used by the ancient Greeks in sacrificial fires or to fumigate and cleanse sacred spaces. Here in North America, the Indigenous people used it for similar purposes and included it in their smudges and fires for protection and purification.

Tree of Life

Another common name for white cedar is arborvitae, meaning the "tree of life" — not to be confused with Yggdrasil, which is an ash tree. This name is fitting, since these trees are among the oldest in North America and the wood, being extremely rot-resistant, can last many seasons on the damp ground. However, this name was likely introduced when early French explorers learned its unique qualities of preventing and curing a disease known as scurvy, and today white cedar is considered to be one of the first Indigenous medicines from North America to be documented.

In the fall of 1535, winter arrived early while Jacques Cartier and his crew were exploring the St. Lawrence River in eastern Canada and his three ships and 110 crew members became trapped in the ice. Within a few weeks, Cartier's men began to suffer from scurvy, which, years later, was determined to be caused from a lack of vitamin C. The symptoms, which include anemia, weakness, hemorrhaging of the skin, bleeding gums and loose teeth, occur quickly if a diet lacks this important nutrient and can be fatal if not treated. By February, eight of Cartier's men were dead and 50 were past the point of recovery. He sought help from the

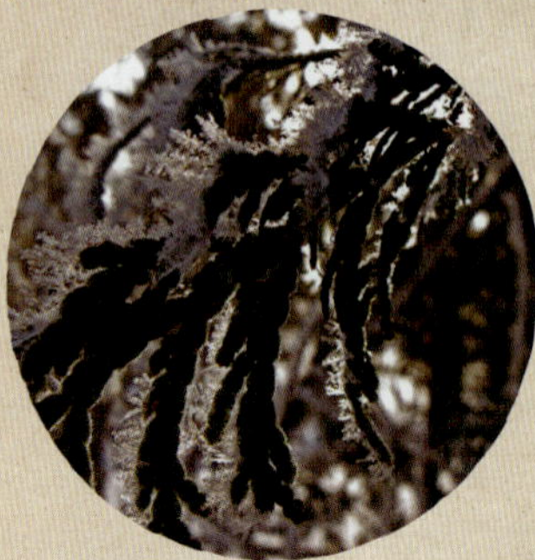

Often referred to as the "tree of life"

Haudenosaunee (Iroquois) people who were camped along the shores. In winter, scurvy was most likely a prevalent disease among the native peoples and the symptoms quite familiar. They showed him how to formulate a remedy by drinking a tea made from the leaves of white cedar (which has been shown to contain vitamin C) and the men recovered quickly. As the story goes, Cartier, or one of his counterparts, took white cedar back to France and presented it to the king, who named it "l'arbor de vie." It was introduced into the Royal Medicine Gardens (Jardin du Roi) in Fontainebleau, France, and became known as arborvitae. White cedar is believed to be one of the first North American trees imported to Europe.

However, there is a small glitch to this story. Cartier never mentioned using cedar, or a tree known as arborvitae, as a remedy that miraculously cures scurvy. Instead, they identified the tree, with remarkable curative abilities, as a very large evergreen known as annedda. Unfortunately, over the years this word has been lost from the native language. Based on documentation by French explorers and the ethno-medicine of Indigenous peoples in eastern Canada, the true identity of arborvitae has become quite controversial. Although today annedda or "tree of life" commonly references white cedar, several other conifers are considered to be good candidates. It has been narrowed down to a handful of trees, including spruce, pine, hemlock and fir, which would have been found along Cartier's travel route near Quebec. These were chosen based on botanical evaluation, naval historical documents, notes from Cartier's contemporaries, folk medicine, and the tree's estimated content of vitamin C. To this day we still do not know the true identity of the tree called annedda and it may be a mystery that is never completely solved.

It wasn't until 1753 that scurvy was recognized by the British medical community as being directly related to a dietary deficiency. By the 1770s, beers prepared from spruce, pines and firs were widely used in Canada to treat the symptoms of scurvy and sold under the name of *sapinette*. When this disease was realized to be a common killer on long sea voyages, these beverages were taken on boats to ensure the health of the crew. Soon after this, it was discovered that citrus fruit contained high amounts of vitamin C, and at the beginning of the nineteenth century it was the practice of the Royal British Navy to add lemon or lime juice to the sailors' daily ration, resulting in some of the healthiest crews of the time. By the 1850s, *lime-juicers*, later shortened to *limeys*, was a derogatory word for sailors in the British Navy.

Wildlife Value

Cedars are also properly named the "tree of life," for wherever there are cedar forests there is also an array of wildlife species. This is evident in winter, when the snow-covered ground beneath them displays a multitude of animal tracks. The fronds that sweep down towards that ground are utilized by a variety of animals for both shelter and browsing. Snowshoe hares, cottontails, porcupines and red squirrels savour the foliage; however, the most ravaging feeders are white tailed deer, with cedars being their most important and preferred winter food. A distinct browse line can be seen on windbreaks or in swamps where deer have pruned them as high as they can reach while standing on their hind legs.

Songbirds also make considerable used of cedar. The seeds support about forty species of birds and cedar-hedges provide valuable habitat. The thick foliage not only supplies a safety zone, it also acts as a heat sink to provide warmth and shelter in winter storms. The fibrous bark offers nesting material for birds and flying squirrels, and branch tips scattered on the ground signify they have been nipped off by red squirrels.

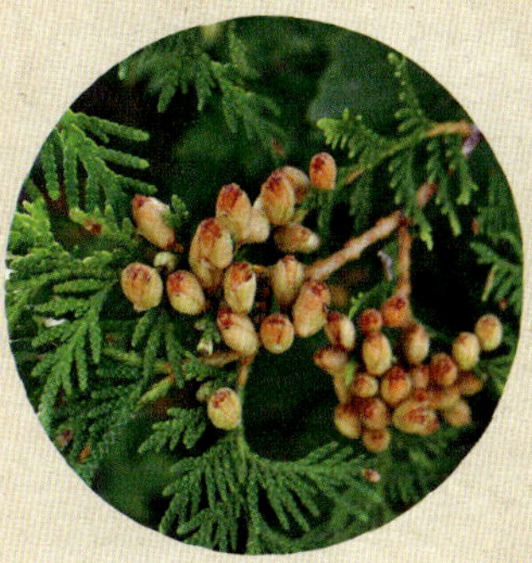

Wildlife treasure cedars for shelter and food

Culinary Uses

Due to the thujone within the plant, cedar is not commonly employed in the kitchen. However, in the past, the leaves and twigs were made into a sweet drink, and the pith in the young shoots was added to soups for its pleasant taste.

Medicinal Uses

North America's First Nations people and nineteenth century eclectic physicians have had a longstanding relationship with this tree, and over the years it has been used for scurvy, rheumatism, warts, sore throats, coughs and to stimulate the uterus. Its main actions are due to its volatile oils, flavonoids and tannins found within the plant. Although the young leafy twigs can be gathered at any time, its medicinal properties are most pronounced when collected in spring or summer.

If used with care, cedar is useful medicine. However, the most active component is the volatile oil known as thujone, a neurotoxin and toxic heart stimulant also found in the banned alcoholic drink absinthe. If used for an appropriate period and in small dosages, cedar is considered safe. Due to its stimulating action on the uterus, it is advisable to avoid it while pregnant.

Warts and Other Skin Issues

The aromatic oils found in the leaves are strongly antifungal, antiviral and antibacterial in action and when applied externally have marked influences on numerous skin afflictions. One of cedar's most unique virtues is its reputation for removing warts, polyps and other skin growths, and its claims are undeniable. It is used with benefit on fungal growths and viral infections, quickly remedying ringworm, athlete's foot, nail fungus, thrush, herpes simplex and cold sores. Make infused oil with the newest green growth and soak or apply it two to four times a day until the issue is resolved. Alternatively, Thuja essential oil, often blended with tea tree oil, can be diluted in castor oil and employed.

Respiratory Complaints

The volatile oils in *Thuja* have been shown to stimulate the immune function by activating certain white blood cells, and work as a bronchodilator to help open the lungs. A leaf decoction, sweetened with honey, has antiviral and antibiotic activities, which is useful for alleviating chronic coughs, sore throats, bronchitis and other signs of respiratory distress. Pulmonary complaints and bronchial catarrh can also be treated through a steam bath. Simmer the foliage in water and pour it into a bowl. With the aid of a towel draped over the head and basin, the vapours are inhaled. Expectorant and decongestant actions are immediate.

Rheumatic Problems

Used with remarkable success, an ointment or compress is excellent for muscular aches, strains, neuralgia, rheumatic pains and arthritis. A folk remedy among the Indigenous people and loggers for generations was to pound the fresh leaves in a mortar and simmer them with fat or oil to make a salve. This mixture was spread on linen and applied to painful joints, giving certain relief. Bathing the afflicted parts in a warm cedar infusion can also play a role in the treatment of rheumatism, and cedar oil continues to have commercial success in the form of medicated rubs.

The Wood

Cedar, along with white birch, is one of the most utilitarian trees in the forest and is held in high regard. Its beautiful, light coloured wood is unlike that of its western cousin red cedar (*Thuja plicata*), which is intensely red. Although it produces little resin, the wood has a sweet smell and it is greatly valued for its many features: incredibly lightweight when dried, easily worked, splits readily, doesn't warp or shrink and resists decay. Commercially, it was once in high demand. "To make up fraite (freight) with other commodities, [it] will yield great profits," is what Thomas Harriot wrote about white cedar in 1590, and ships returning to England from Virginia carried cargoes of cedar wood. It grew plentifully in Canada, and by 1880 cedar was being sold for fence posts, railway ties, telegraph poles and light roofing timber in Ontario and Quebec for $16 to $20 per thousand feet.

Cedar is extremely rot-resistant and long-lasting when coming in contact with soil and moisture, due to its natural antifungal properties. Because of its perpetual nature, it provides ideal wood for fencing and shingles. Cedar rail fences once snaked all over our countryside, and Canadian naturalist Gosse noted in 1840 that the "facility with which it is split, but chiefly from its great durability, almost incorruptibility, it is in great request for the rails that compose zigzag fences." He went on to say that cedar rails "may be exposed to every vicissitude of weather for a man's lifetime without manifesting any symptoms of decay." Almost a hundred years earlier, naturalist Peter Kalm also mentioned cedar being the most commonly used wood for fencing and wrote, "Since it is thought the most durable in Canada and that which best withstands rotting, so as to remain undamaged for over a man's age, fences of all kinds are scarcely made of any other then this wood." Another characteristic of cedar wood is that it splits and separates easily along its annual growth rings (a feature known as ring shake), making it the wood of choice for wooden shingles and shakes for house and barn roofs.

Owing to the fact that cedar wood does not shrink or warp, the Native Americans used this tree for their cedar strip canoes and the frames and ribs of their birchbark canoes. In 1613, Champlain, who at the time was on the Ottawa River, wrote, "Their canoes are made of birch bark reinforced with little circles of cedar wood very well arranged." These same people would occasionally substitute cedar bark for white birch bark to cover their lodges or to make containers. They also used the wood for their ceremonial drums, traditional fishing spears and other cultural artwork.

Fires

Not only does cedar have a gift for generating warmth by blocking the wind and trapping and storing heat in its foliage, it provides excellent fuel for fires, since the wood readily burns and is easy to ignite. Perhaps because of these features, this tree has had a long connection with the element of fire and the sun. The wood is used in bow drills to start fires by friction, and the bark is shredded into "nests" in which to throw the sparks. Although they initiate lots of crackling and popping, even the fresh, green fronds will burn with great ease, getting the fire roaring.

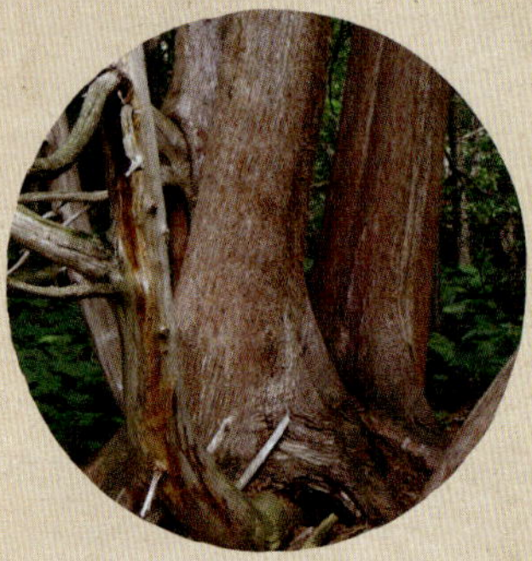

The wood is rot resistant and does not shrink or warp

Incense, Smudges and Sweat Lodges

The essential oils in the leaves are commonly used in the perfume industry. As well, the wood is a major ingredient in making incense and when ground into a fine powder and burned, it yields a pleasing, woodsy fragrance. Its balsamic smell is calming to the senses, and aromatherapist Jeanne Rose noted it is "useful in smoothing transition and grieving loss, which may cause both emotional and physical disharmonies of the heart."

The dried leaves are used in the traditional smudging sticks of the North American Indigenous people, where during ceremonies it is customary to purify sacred objects and the people participating with cedar smoke. This cleanses negative energy, creates a sacred space and puts one in a proper state of mind. Cedar is also extensively used in sweat lodges to purify and strengthen the spirit.

Other Uses

As early as the 1600s, it was recorded that early Canadians used cedar to make brooms. In 1749, botanist Peter Kalm in Quebec wrote of cedar, "Its branches are used all over Canada for brooms and the twigs and leaves of it being naturally bent together seem to be very proper for this purpose." As well, because of its pleasing scent, the fresh branches were used as a besom sweep, a practice of the ancient Celts. These sweeps of fresh green boughs not only helped rid the home of pests and vermin; they also cleared any negative influences.

Legends and Myths

Cedar is featured in many legends. Its trait of crackling, popping and liberating sparks while burning seems to have been a major theme. A fawn got its spots when mother deer placed her young beside a fire of cedar to keep it warm and the ashes gently landed on its back, leaving beautiful snow-white markings. The sparks that floated up into the heavens were believed to have created the stars that flicker in the sky. Magical flutes were also made of cedar wood. A young man who played the flute would instinctively know what game to hunt and where to find it. If the instrument was made from wood that had been stuck by lightning, it was believed to have influential powers for wooing a woman.

Folklore

Cedar was thought to afford infallible protection. Burning the fragrant wood provided a pleasing smell and acted as a powerful guardian against diseases and negative influences. If a cedar took root on your property, it was imperative that it not be cut. As long as it flourished, your family would have good health and your home would be protected from harmful forces. Cedar was also associated with prayers and divine alignment, and was used to help summon helpful spirits during rituals and religious ceremonies.

Due to its durability and resistance to rot, cedar became linked with longevity and preservation. It was given eternal status and frequently carried as a talisman to inspire a prosperous and healthy life. The wood was burned at baby rituals to bring it a long life, and newborns were washed in a warm cedar infusion before presenting them to the community. As a tree of immortality, it was used at funerals and planted around cemeteries for its evergreen qualities and symbolism for eternal life. It represents unchanging friendship, and in the *Language of Flowers,* it means "I live but for thee."

Lessons of Cedar

Grandmother cedar holds old wisdom and strength that can assist in healthy spiritual growth. When standing within her protective embrace, she heals us from trauma and suffering and can even help you become invisible should the need arise. She is a symbol of generosity and represents integrity, kindness and righteousness.

White Pine

Pinus strobus

Wind Tree, Whispering Pine, Weymouth Pine, Knotty Pine, Northern Pine, Soft Pine

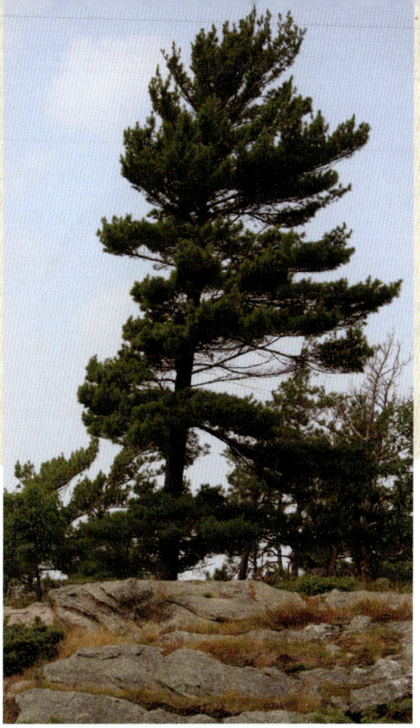

White pine is fittingly named "wind tree." This title is twofold. First, it refers to the airy and divine quality of the tree as the soft, flexible needles instill calmness, tranquility and serenity. When the wind blows through their boughs, it is thought to whisper messages from the heavens. White pine forests, therefore, are sacred places that should be approached and entered in reverence in order to be respectful to the spirits living within. Because of its alleged ability to pick up voices in the breeze, in songs and poems it became romantically known as the "whispering pine."

Secondly, white pine is capable of enduring harsh environments, especially along Northern Ontario's rocky shores. On these unprotected landscapes, exposed trees become stunted and windswept, and their picturesque silhouettes have been made famous by Canadian artists, particularly a collection of painters known as The Group of Seven.

The Monarch of the Forest

Considered the monarch of Canadian forests, this tree's majestic stature is a sight to behold as it reaches into the heavens. When Europeans first arrived on the shores of North America, they were greeted with pines that routinely reached heights of 45 to 60 meters (150 to 200 feet). White pine is deemed the largest conifer east of the Rockies. Claims were made that its height was so impressive that at night, the stars in the sky hung from its great branches.

White pine is considered a super-canopy tree, towering over other species in the forest. Not only do these lofty trees play an important role as nesting sites and landmarks

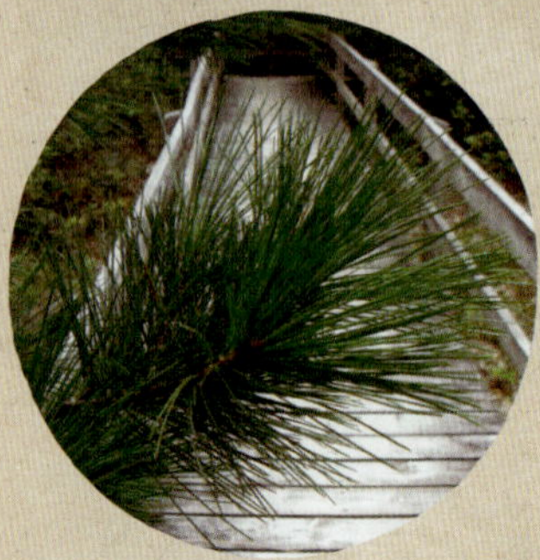

The needles are soft when brushed against the skin

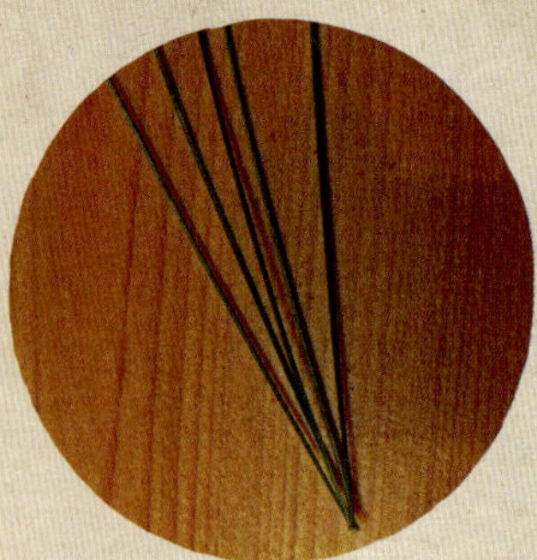

The pliable needles are in bundles of five

for our owls and hawks, they were deemed sacred because these birds of prey, perched on top of the tree, sounded an alarm if danger was imminent. Furthermore, due to its height, ancient cultures believed this tree could see great distances to far-off horizons, and it was considered an asset for assisting with long sight, clear vision and understanding of what is beyond and yet to come.

Meeting White Pine

A certain stillness can be found while walking among pines, and anyone who wants peace of mind, protection or shelter can find refuge beneath their boughs. In old-growth forests, this truly magnificent tree lives to be 450 years or older, holding great knowledge and wisdom from the past. Today, however, due to its high lumber value, most are cut before they reach the prime of their life. On summer days their volatile oils are released into the atmosphere and the aroma can evoke childhood memories of times spent playing among the pines on rocky outcrops or camping trips with family. For others, the scent is associated with Christmas, as this beautiful tree is frequently used during holiday celebrations.

Due to its grace and charm, white pine is valued in garden settings. The evergreen needles allow its beauty to last through the seasons and add life to drab winter landscapes when other plants are dormant. The wind, amplified through its needles, sounds like a babbling brook, and the soft foliage just beg to have fingers run through them. The scent from the tree calms the nerves and provokes relaxation, while at the same time elevating the spirit and clearing the mind.

Evergreen Needles

White pine is easily identified. It is the only pine east of the Rockies that carries its pliable needles in bundles of five. The needles are soft to the touch and the entire tree has a feathery, elegant appearance. Though the tree retains green foliage throughout the year, the needles don't remain forever. After the inner needles reach the end of their second year, they start to discolour and fall to the ground, forming a soft carpet underfoot. This yellowing occurs annually and is a natural process in the tree's life cycle.

As the tree grows upward, new branches form a complete ring around the trunk. Since each ensuing whorl represents a year of the tree's life, an approximate age can be determined by counting the layers of branches. As the tree matures, however, it loses its lower branches, making this aging technique inaccurate. Noting the distance between the whorls can help analyze its past growing seasons. Large gaps signify good growing conditions, whereas a relatively shorter space indicates an environmental hardship, such as drought. Comparing the growth patterns with surrounding trees helps determine whether a general or individual setback occurred.

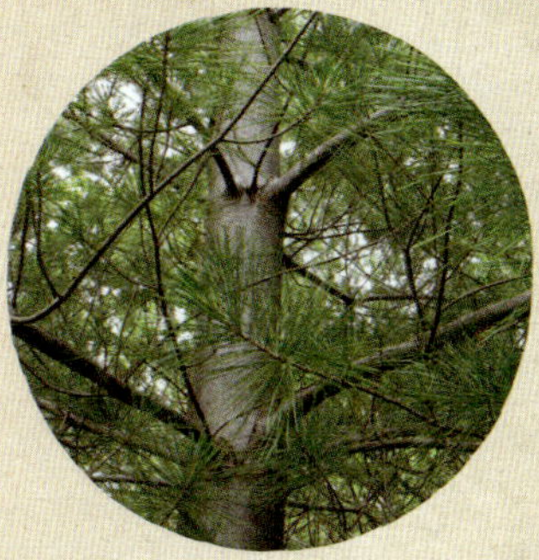

A whorl of branches represents each year of life

Pine Cones

A light breeze is important for the reproductive cycle of the wind tree. Male and female flowers develop on the same tree and rely on wind pollination. In dry weather the male flowers release vast quantities of sulfur-yellow pollen into the air for it to be received by the female flowers situated at the tips of new shoots high in the crown. Once the female cone is fertilized, it closes up tight and remains sealed until the seeds fully ripen. It takes two summers for the cones to develop, and when mature, the dry, woody scales open to release the winged seeds. These, too, are carried off in the wind to be dispersed to new locations. It is possible then to find three generations of cones on the same tree: the newly forming cones from the current year, the tightly sealed cones with fertilized seeds from the previous year;

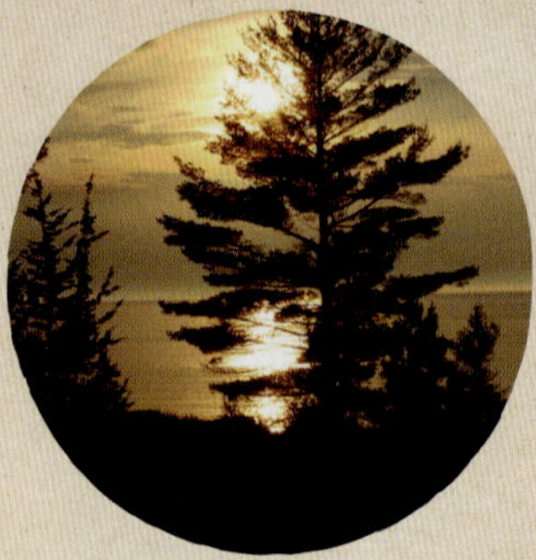

White pine is known as the "Tree of Peace"

and old, spent cones that have shed their seeds to the wind from two years before.

In many European cultures, pine cones symbolized fertility (especially female fertility) and were used during the Spring Equinox festival to increase the fruitfulness of the land.

The "Tree of Peace"

When the Mohawk, Oneida, Onondaga, Cayuga and Seneca tribes residing on land that is now the state of New York grew tired of fighting, the chiefs agreed to meet and formed the Iroquois or Haudenosaunee Confederacy. It was the white pine that came to symbolize this union; the five tribes joined together as one, like the five needles joined together on white pine branches. It became known as the "Tree of Peace" and still carries great power in their tradition. At the time, the chiefs buried their weapons beneath a giant pine, where they were carried away by underground waters, and the roots, extending in all four directions, were called "roots of peace." This ancient tree was to represent the passing of this "Great Peace" from those first chiefs to their children, keeping the promise alive long after they died. The spirit of the original tree lives in the hearts of the people when they gather in pine forests today. They are continually reminded that weapons of war should be cast aside and harmony should be preserved. Spending time with white pine helps facilitate peace among friends, family and community and reminds us to love others and embrace our differences.

Association with Springtails

We have all heard of insectivorous plants that trap insects to convert them into plant nutrients. Now it appears that some plants can get nitrogen from insects through a fungal relationship. Soil ecologists John Klironomos and Miranda Hat at the University of Guelph in Ontario, Canada, have recently discovered that white pines get some of their nitrogen from a carnivorous fungus, bicolored deceiver (*Laccaria bicolor*), which is able to kill tiny soil arthropods called springtails (*Folsomia candida*). Though barely visible, springtails are essential members of the community; they play a key role in recycling nutrients and making soil by helping fragment organic material so that it is easier for decomposers to break down.

Bicolored deceiver grows around tree roots and sends out filaments into the soil in search of water and mineral to pass onto the trees. However, it is now understood that they also seek out springtails. When the soil is lacking in nitrogen, the fungus is able to paralyze and ingest springtails using special enzymes, thereby releasing additional nitrogen tied up in the arthropod's bodies. Pine trees have partnered up with these fungi so that these nutrients are transferred to their roots in exchange for sugars produced during photosynthesis.

This fungal association has changed how science looks at nutrient cycling in forests. In plant nutrition, science has long recognized the importance of partnerships between trees and ectomycorrhizal fungi (fungi that grow on tree roots). Until now, however, it was believed that trees and their associated fungi obtained nitrogen from microbial decomposition of dead organic matter and nitrogen-fixing bacteria; not feasting on live animals like springtails.

Wildlife Value

Numerous species of animals love the safe and peaceful presence of white pine. The large branches and crotches make excellent nesting sites that offer safety and cover for birds. Broad winged, sharp shinned and cooper's hawks begin their courtship and nest building in early spring. Some return to previous nests and refurbish them with fresh sprigs, or owls adopt them for their own use. Other animals will also use white pine for habitat; deer rest beneath the boughs, raccoons employ them for daytime sleeping spots, and red squirrels use the soft twigs as bedding material.

While the evergreen boughs provide shelter, conifers rot from the outside and rarely make adequate cavity trees for animals to dwell inside. Declining trees, however, harbor plenty of insects, affording excellent feeding sites for woodpeckers. Even fallen logs are not lost and offer valued habitat for ring-necked snakes and salamanders. Due to the high resin content, pine wood is slow to decompose, and a large log can last over a hundred years on the forest floor.

White pine also offers sustenance for a variety of animals. Pine needles themselves provide a meal to butterfly and moth larvae, and birds feed their young on these caterpillars. The winged seeds are food for many birds and small mammals and red squirrels store caches of cones, known as middens, at the base of trees. They can quickly strip a cone of its seeds, and a pile of bare cones and discarded scales indicates red squirrel activity. Although grey squirrels are not big consumers of the seeds, they do play an important role in the life cycle of pines. Studies have found that the act of burying acorns and other nuts encourages pine germination by providing bare seedbeds, and pine seedlings tend to be in greater abundance beneath oaks and hickories when grey squirrels are active.

Culinary Uses

Almost every part of this tree can be consumed, providing emergency food throughout the year. The young needles make a pleasant tea and are rich in vitamin C. Early settlers and Indigenous people used the needles to boost their immunity in order to survive the long, harsh winters and to prevent scurvy, which affected many voyagers after months at sea with limited diets. In spring, the new shoots, when stripped of their needles and peeled, can be candied by simmering them in sugary syrup. Also in spring, the sweetish, inner bark is edible and was once dried and ground into nutritious flour. The young cones, when boiled, were eaten, while the protein-rich pollen from the male flower was used to thicken stews, enrich cereals, or combined with other flours to make breads and cakes. The unopened cones were heated to roast and release the seeds and then ground into meal or mixed with dried berries for storage. Some species have big seeds, and the most commonly sold pine nut in supermarkets today is from the Colorado pinyon pine (*Pinus edulis*).

Medicinal Uses

White pine is a tree that provides valuable medicine. Most commonly, it is used to ease breathing disorders, treat skin complaints and alleviate rheumatic pain. Its healing effects are, in part, due to its aromatic resinous oils and tannins, which are antiseptic to the lungs, skin and urinary tract.

To harvest, remove the inner bark from the branches in early spring and decoct it slowly to release the medicinal properties. Alternatively, steep the freshly picked needles in water for 12 to 24 hours to use as a base for cough syrup, or make a salve from the pitch. Like all herbs, when harvesting, it is customary to leave a gift as an offering to the plant.

Respiratory Tract

White pine is useful for facilitating breathing, thinning and loosening phlegm, relieving spasms and fighting germs. As an aromatic antimicrobial, it has the ability to directly kill germs while exerting an opening action on the lungs. It helps fight infections in the respiratory tract and is employed at the onset of colds and flus to prevent them from moving deep into the lungs. At the same time, its expectorant properties help relieve congestion by thinning and drawing up mucus so that it is easier to eliminate. A tea from the needles and inner bark can be used to treat respiratory complaints such as bronchitis, spasmodic coughs, colds, sore throats, asthma and other breathing difficulties. The resin is also used in cough syrups and, when inhaled in a steam pot or applied as a chest compress, it helps break up catarrh.

Walking Through Pines

Since the aromatic oils are readily released into the air, simply walking through a mature forest is beneficial to one's health. In fact, pine-forest retreats were once used as an aid in the treatment of tuberculosis and other consumptive diseases. For this reason, people traveled many miles to lie under their boughs. Parents were advised to take an ailing child to where pines were plentiful so its aroma could be inhaled daily. It is deemed healthy to have them growing near dwellings, since breathing in the volatile oils enhances immunity, improves circulation in the capillary beds of the lungs and increases oxygen uptake in the cells. In addition, the phenols contained in pine oil also act as a natural stress reliever, making this tree popular in aromatherapy.

Treating Wounds

The resin, which flows from the tree, is antimicrobial, mildly antifungal and anti-inflammatory. In the tree, its role is to help seal tree wounds and offer protection against insects, fungi and other infestations. When employed topically to the skin, however, it disinfects wounds, draws out infection and reduces swelling. Most notably, it escalates foreign-body responses by provoking an increase in white blood cells, which results in a faster healing time. This influence makes it especially valuable for neglected wounds that have become putrid.

In *The Herball, or Generall Historie of Plantes*, published in 1597, herbalist and botanist John Gerard (1545-1612) claimed pine salve was a sovereign remedy for wounds and wrote, “out of pine trees there issueth a liquid, whitish and sweet-smelling rosin very aptly mixed in ointment for the commanded healing up of wounds.” It has been used for centuries to disinfect and seal up wounds, and to draw out debris, infections and other unwanted impurities from the body. It was particularly beneficial as a dressing to bring boils to a head and pull-out embedded splinters and thorns. It was suggested that it successfully treated gunshot wounds, even after gangrene had set in. Today pine salve is still found on fishing boats to help draw out stubborn slivers painlessly.

Rheumatic Pain

Pine is a classic remedy to ease joint pain and inflammation. When the essential oil is added to massage oil or put in a bath, it improves circulation, relaxes sore muscles and relieves chronic rheumatism, arthritis and neuralgia. Alternatively, pine oil can be made by simply covering the needles or pitch with good quality oil and leaving it in the oven on low heat (180 degrees F) overnight to release the healing properties.

Valuable Lumber

White pines were so abundant when Europeans first landed on the shores of North America, they professed that a squirrel could travel through these forests its entire life without setting a paw on the ground. The timber from this iconic tree soon became well-known around the world, and economically, it became an important tree in Canadian history. Growing to amazing heights and sizes, it was not uncommon to see logs 120 feet long and 4 feet in diameter. To get these huge logs to the mills, Canadian lumberjacks floated them down rivers in log drives. These scenes were commemorated in paintings, stories, poems and songs like “The Log Drivers Waltz.”

Ship Building

The tall, straight trunks of white pine were highly valued and particularly ideal for making masts for sailing vessels; so much so that they were declared a national treasure. At the time, there was a deficit of such lumber in Europe, and to make up for the shortfall, the British Navy constructed inferior masts by piecing together Scots pines. Once their main masts were made from our white pine, the British Royal Navy soon formed one of the most powerful fleets of ships in the world. Every year, representatives of the king would select the tallest and straightest pines and mark them with a symbol known as the "King's Broad Arrow." The symbols meant that these trees were reserved for the Crown and that early settlers could not cut them for their own use. White pine became Ontario's official tree in 1984 and was given this designation because it played such an important role in the timber industry.

Because it is easily worked and the high resin content in the wood slows decay, pine has been employed in boat building since the time of early Greece. In fact, some speculate that the botanical name *Pinus* may have been derived from an old term for boat or raft. Craftsmen advised not to fell a pine tree for ship building during the waning of the moon, as the moon was said to influence the resin content of the wood, making it less sea worthy. Some old-timers still believe this to be true today.

The "Tree that Built North America"

In the eighteenth and nineteenth centuries, white pine supported almost the entire timber industry, and was dubbed the "tree that built North America." Due to its soft, strong, workable qualities, it was extensively used by the pioneers to construct their homes and all their furniture. Their chests, sideboards, bedsteads, tables and cupboards are now highly sought after by antique dealers and are known as primitive furniture. So large were the boards, a three-foot-wide table could be made from a single piece of clean wood. The lumber could be found in a variety of things such as coffins, covered bridges, boardwalks, bobsleds, and musical instruments. Even today, white pine remains one of our most valuable construction materials and is commonly used for door frames, window sashes, moulding and trim. The wood is frequently referred to as "knotty pine" due to the knots that form from the dead, lower branches still attached to the trunk. Some woodworkers consider this a fault that weakens the wood, while others claim it adds character to the piece.

The Resin

The specific name *strobus* signifies a tree that yields an odoriferous gum or is "incense-bearing." This name points to other products obtained from white pine, such as pitch, turpentine and rosin. Historically, pitch was made by slowly heating resinous bark, cones and chunks of wood in pits, straining it through a filter and then packing it into containers. The thick, tarry substance could then be reheated to the proper consistency and used for glue, caulking, waterproofing and as a protective coating. Once applied, a fine layer of white ash from a fire was sprinkled on the gooey substance, which then became hard enough to sand smooth. It was used to line beer barrels, fill cracked pots, and seal boats and canoes. The Greeks smeared pine pitch on the inside of clay vessels used to hold their wine. This yielded a distinctive resinous flavour to the wine for which they called Retsina. To this day, Retsina is still made with pine resin to give it an authentic flavour.

The practice of sealing ships with pine pitch is very ancient, and in the Bible God instructed Noah to "cover the ark, within and without, with pitch" (Genesis 6:14). First Nations people used the gum to mend and cover the seams of their birchbark canoes. The largest consumer of pine pitch and tar however, was the British navy, which used it for caulking their vessels and to waterproof wood, rope and canvas. This is why, since the seventeenth century, their sailors have been referred to as "tars."

Rosin, which is precipitated from crude resin, is brittle when dry and sticky when heated. Baseball players rub it on their bats for a better hold and violinists apply it to their bow to obtain better string grip and enhance vibration. After the rosin is removed, turpentine is distilled from the liquid left over. This is often used as a cleaning agent for oil-based paints. The most expensive resin product, however, is amber. This golden jewel is fossilized resin from extinct pines and holds the distinction of being the only jewel of plant origin.

Other Uses

In England and Scotland, twice a year, pails of smouldering needles were brought into houses to rid them of fleas and other pests and to prevent diseases. Today, pine is still often used in insecticides, air fresheners and cleaning products, due to its fresh scent and disinfectant qualities. It is also a common addition to perfumes, and the sawdust is often used as a base for incenses. The cones can be used as tinder for fires, children's crafts and for pet bunnies to play and gnaw on.

Yule Celebration

Because pines remain green throughout the year, they were thought to possess the essence of divine being and to symbolize light and renewed life. During the Midwinter festival of Yule, the ancient Druids made large bonfires of pine to celebrate the changing of the seasons and help draw back the

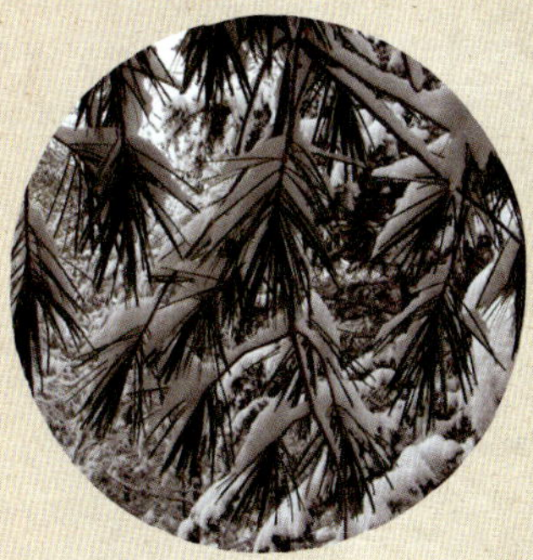

The evergreen needles add life to drab winter landscapes

sun. In the same way, the boughs were made into wreaths and garlands and brought into homes as a reminder of the eternal energy force and the promise of continued life. Pine trees themselves were decorated with lights and shiny objects to encourage light to triumph over darkness. These pagan traditions are still celebrated today during the Christmas season as Yule logs, Christmas wreaths, and Christmas trees, which now represent hope, God's everlasting love and the light of Christ.

Longevity and Immortality

In a similar way, these evergreen trees were a powerful symbol of immortality. Pine trees were planted in cemeteries or the boughs placed on graves to remind the living that life is eternal. The wood is often used in coffins, and the needles are burned to bring encouragement and healing to the bereaved. Taken as an elixir, pine promotes longevity, and carrying the cone was thought to impart vigor in old age.

Birth

Pine is a feminine tree. It is one of the primary birthing trees sacred to the Greek goddess Artemis, who presided over the moon and childbirth. Pines are often established to commemorate new beginnings, renewal of life or the start of an era. In northern cultures, a pine seed was planted at the birth of a new child to symbolize that all great things grow from small seeds.

Joy, Peace and Blessings

Pine groves are thought of as benevolent places where people can rest safely in the protective aura of the trees. They are calming and uplifting, bringing both joy and a deep sense of inner peace. It was believed that fairies, angels and kind spirits live among the boughs, and branches were tied to doors in hopes of attracting them. It was customary to plant two pines in front of dwellings to bring healing energy, continuous joy and blessings to the family within. They are also places to hang one's burdens before entering the

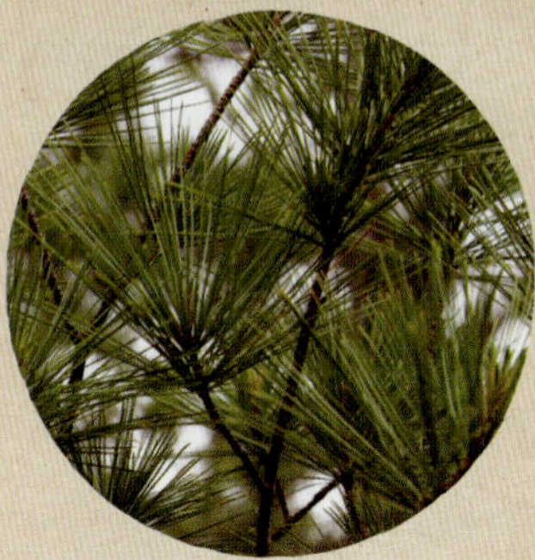

The evergreen boughs are a promise of continued life

home and being with family.

Banishes Negativity

According to the Celts, pine fairies were solitary beings that had a healing presence and encouraged positive energy. Hanging pine branches over doors and windows or scattering the needles on the floor was rumoured to prevent evil from entering the building while at the same time bringing a peaceful energy. Throwing the needles and cones into winter fires protected the hearth and home and removed negative influences. Brooms or besoms made from pine boughs sanctified and purified gardens and new homes, and pine oil in wash water eliminated unwanted spirits (most likely in the form of germs). Farmers also transferred pine's evergreen vitality and protective powers to barns by sweeping them with pine brooms and hanging the branches on stable doors.

Folklore

Since pine cones grow in a spiral shape, they were thought to be good conductors of magical energy, especially when gathered on the Summer Solstice. Connected with abundance, the cones were believed to bestow good fortune and prosperity to the holder, and could attract gold or draw in a steady income. Some ancient cultures believed that pines held the mysteries and secrets of fire, which they guarded closely, while others associated pine with the rain and burned the cones in hopes of bringing favourable weather.

The Celts also believed that the smoke offered their prayers a ride to heaven and that any wishes would be granted if spoken from the heart. Another belief proclaimed that eating one pine nut from a cone every day would provide protection from gun shots.

Lessons of White Pine

Pine has a special connection with light, the sun and life on earth. Its energy can awaken the light within us, and nurturing it to grow inspires us to keep our internal spark alive by embracing every day and living in the present. It can help us see the bright side of situations: when things look hopeless, we can choose to stay in the dark, feeling afraid, or we can move to the light and bask in the sunshine.

A walk in a pine grove brings insight and deeper contemplation, giving you a new perspective on a situation or problem. The pines' lofty height encourages farsightedness and urges one to broaden one's horizons. This outlook inspires us to rise above difficult times, overcoming hardships and persisting against all odds. It helps us find our purpose in life by setting our feet upon the earth and pointing the way to see a clear path forward. This allows us to stay the course so that we can emerge with a renewed sense of purpose.

In Bach's flower remedies, pine is said to release guilt and self-blame. It helps liberate negativity, unhealthy thoughts we are holding onto, and provides support so we don't dwell on past mistakes or assign blame. Just as it draws out splinters, infections and other unwanted substances from the body, pine can pull out old pain and festering wounds to let peace flow within. As the wind blows up new prospects, it allows you leave the past behind. Pine shows us it is enough just to be and dance in the wind.

Willow

Salix spp.

Swamp Tree, Sallow, Saille, Osier, Withy, Witches' Aspirin, Witches' Tree, Tree of Witcheries and Tree of Enchantment

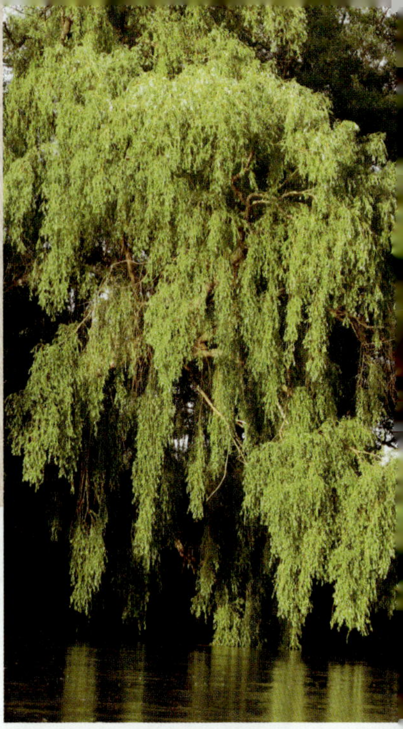

Even in the bleak winter landscape, willow holds bright yellow branches, ensuring that all take notice. This water-loving tree thrives in damp soils along streams and rivers prone to flooding, and in the past signified a reliable water source for thirsty travelers. Because willow seeks locations close to water, it was commissioned as the guardian of watersheds. The graceful branches that gently sway in the wind are often seen hanging over river banks, and it is here that willow reigns as queen. When canoeing, I make a special effort to paddle under the drooping boughs, for it is said that this tree has a healing aura and blesses all those it touches. It was honoured by the Druids and is one of the seven sacred trees of the Irish.

The Tree of Water and Moon

Willow not only represents water but also the moon, and this theme is reflected in many stories and legends. The tidal movements of the sea are governed by the moon, and rain is considered a precious gift given by her; therefore, willow is her tree. Even in his *Complete Herbal*, Nicholas Culpeper stated "the moon owns the willow." It brings the energy of water and the moon's blessings into our life and can put us in touch with our deeper feelings and emotions. Willow leaves were traditionally worn during spring celebration or lunar rituals and the wood was fashioned into magic wands especially dedicated to water and moon magic. Due to willow's association with water and moon enchantments, it was revered by rainmakers.

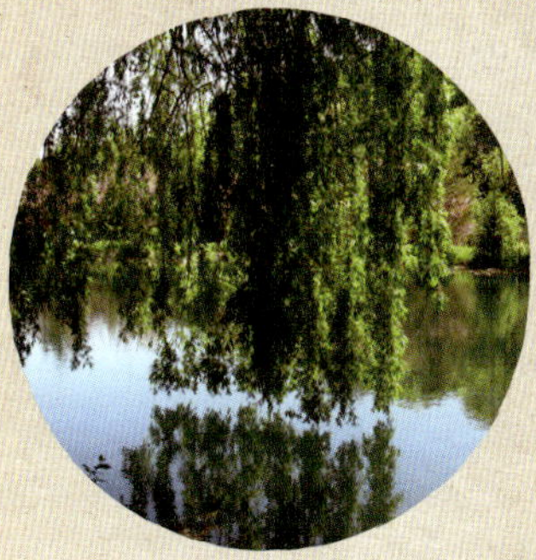

Willow is the tree of the moon, water and women's mysteries

Women's Mysteries

Willow is also the tree of women, representing feminine mystery and lunar rhythms of life, and can help reveal our feminine side to bring spiritual balance. Celtic women held it in high regard for its nurturing aspect and ability to provide intuitive wisdom and insight into nature and its workings. It represents the three aspects of the goddess: lithe and supple like the maiden, fertile like the mother and wise like the crone.

Meeting Willow

Flooding and silting do not seem to inconvenience willows; however, they won't tolerate shade, and for this reason they are usually found growing as solitary trees or in even-aged stands. Although fast-growing, they are relatively short-lived, maturing in about fifty years. There is an old saying, "When a willow grows enough to cast a grave-size shadow, a family member will die."

The silky, silvery-gray catkins of the pussy willow (*Salix discolor*) are admired by children young and old. How they came to be is told in this story. Early one spring, three kittens fell into the river. Upon hearing their cries, willow bent its graceful branches into the water and caught them as they were being swept away in the current. The kittens were brought safely to shore, and now every spring, furry buds emerge at the branch tips where the kittens held on.

One of my first memories of willow was venturing out in spring with my grandmother, who was an avid floral designer, to cut pussy willow branches for her arrangements. She once recited this nursery rhyme to me:

I know a little pussy,
her coat is silver grey
She lives down in the mead-
ow, not very far away

The male and female flowers develop separately, and the furry catkins on pussy willow are the male flowers—not female, as the poem implies—and laden with pollen. Both emerge on naked branches, offering the first hint of spring. After wind or insect pollination, the seeds begin

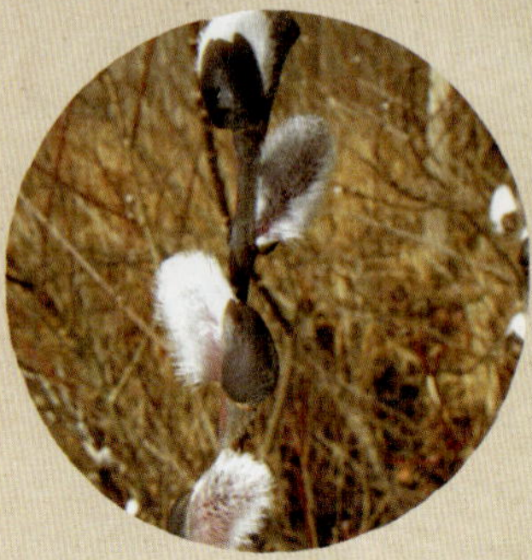

The silver-gray catkins of pussy willow

to develop and are equipped with silky plumes. Although plenty of seeds are produced, they tend to quickly lose their viability.

Prolific Rooters

Willows are enthusiastic reproducers, and the young branches, which are easily broken in wind and ice storms, sprout readily if deposited on muddy banks. Most get their start in life from one of these cast-off twigs, accounting for willow's widespread distribution along watercourses. They often occupy the concave or outer curves of the rivers where the twigs have been washed or pushed to shore by the water's action.

This remarkable ability to sprout from cuttings is attributed to a natural growth hormone present within the plant, which stimulates the development of roots. What is more amazing is that willows are willing to share this gift with other plants, and nursery owners have taken advantage of this trait. When the leaves and bark are chopped and soaked in water, the water-soluble hormone is released into the liquid. Treating cuttings to a drink of willow infusion encourages them to root more willingly.

Because their cuttings readily root, this makes willow useful for bioengineering projects. The fibrous roots function to stabilize banks, thereby controlling erosion along vulnerable waterways during flooding and storm events. However, they can be the bane of city engineers and farmers, since their traveling roots will search out and create havoc in water pipes, drainage tiles and septic systems.

Because of its remarkable ease of quickly sprouting from cuttings or fallen branches, willow symbol-

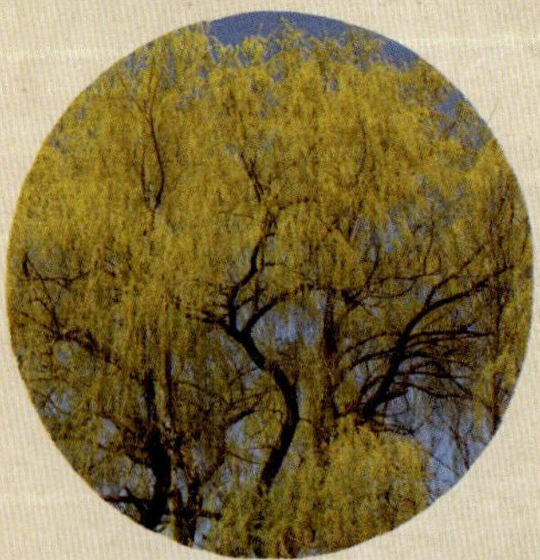

The bark holds rooting hormones

izes renewed growth, vitality and immortality. Christian missionaries carried willow staffs and casually stuck them in the ground, where they dramatically took root and grew, impressing the unconverted. In Great Britain, Christian churches carry willow boughs (called "palm willows") on Palm Sunday instead of palm fronds to symbolize the palms strewn before Jesus as he entered Jerusalem.

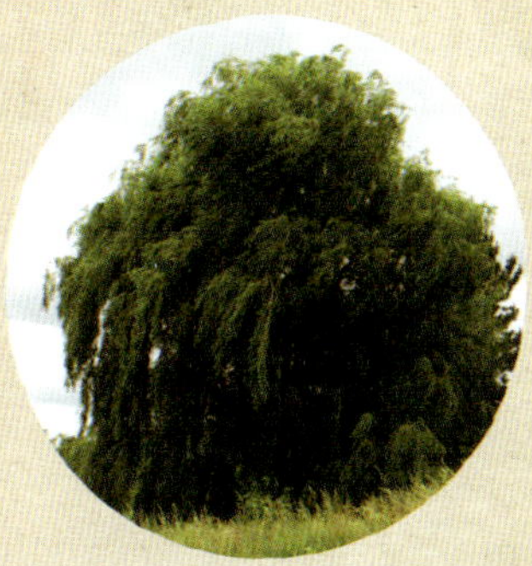

The weeping form brings a peaceful atmosphere to the landscape

In the Garden

Willows come in all shapes and sizes and are widely used in the landscape trade. The long, elegant leaves are among the first to flush in spring, and bright yellow foliage graces the tree in fall. The supple branches add colour to the garden through the dreary winter months, showing hues of bright yellow, red or purple, with the pigment intensifying as spring approaches. Probably the most beloved willow is the golden weeping willow (*Salix babylonica*), which has been adopted in gardens throughout the world. This iconic tree is prized for its elegant beauty and for bringing a relaxing, peaceful atmosphere to the landscape.

Wildlife Value

During winter, there is plenty of evidence of cottontails, hares, muskrats and porcupines gnawing the branches, and in summer they feast on the leaves. Deer, elk and moose browse the foliage and tender twigs; grouse and squirrels nibble the buds; and, along with poplar, willows are a favourite of beavers. Moreover, shrub willows are prolific growers, creating dense thickets near rivers and wetlands, and are not only useful for children playing hide and seek,

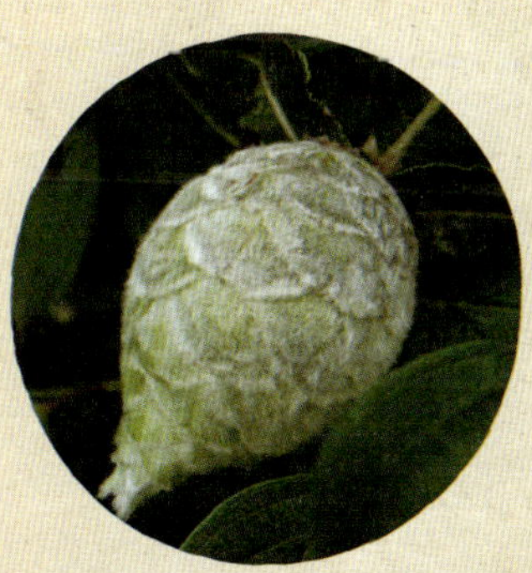

Pinecone willow gall

but also provide excellent nesting sites for song birds. The cottony seeds are soft and warm, making suitable material for lining nests. When concealed in the foliage, the cascading tree branches offer birds shelter, refuge from predators and roosting sites at night.

In early spring, the catkins are abuzz with bees and other flying visitors. Rich in both nectar and pollen, this is one of the first food sources for early pollinators and often their lifeline after enduring the cold winter. There are a number of showy butterflies and moths that use willows as a host plant. The hungry caterpillars of tortoise shells, mourning cloaks, viceroys, white admirals, red-spotted purples and several sphinx moths devour the foliage. These in turn are consumed by birds and are especially valuable for feeding their nestlings, which require a high-protein diet for growth.

Several gall gnats make their homes on willow branches, often being mistaken for cones or seed pods. These gall formations become more prevalent in winter and are created from the plant's response to larvae feeding in the shoot tips. One common gall is the pinecone willow gall, whose cone-like shape and overlapping scales suggest a seed cone.

Meaning of its Name

Willow's trait of thriving along streams and rivers is reflected in the genus name Salix, which was derived from the Celtic word *sal-lis*, meaning "to be near water" or "she is water seeking." This association with water brought about other common names, such as "sallow" and "swamp tree." Likewise, the Celtic word for willow is *saille*. This was anglicized to "sally," meaning a sudden outburst of emotions, actions or expression, as in to "sally forth." This reflects the underlying energy or spirit of willow, which belongs to spring, when all life is stirring with a resurgent of regrowth.

The origin of *willow* has an interesting history. While some say the name came from the Anglo-Saxon word *welig*, meaning soft and pliable, likely referencing the flexible branches, others claim it came from the word *wic*. Wics were communities in rural areas of Europe that, instead of being self-sufficient, growing food, making clothing and creating tools only for themselves, had the distinction of providing surplus produce, crafts and other desired materials to surrounding communities. These villages became known as centers of specialized trades, where commodities and crafts were sold, including honey, cheese, ale, metalwork, woodwork, textiles, pottery and leatherwork. Perhaps because of their skills, people that practiced these old country ways were referred to as *wiccans*, which referred to those who had the ability to manipulate and bend raw material into useful products. Through the years, this evolved into the idea of witchcraft and Wicca, a pagan lifestyle, and bending became related to magic, spells, and manipulating situations or bending other's will. Thus, it has been suggested that willow, wicker, Wiccan and witch are all derived from the same root, meaning to bend.

Willow is sometimes referred to as *withy* or *osier* due to the fact that the slender, pliable branches are suitable for weaving. Its medicinal properties, which were beloved by hedge witches for their gifts of healing, brought about the names witches' tree, witches' aspirin and tree of witcheries. Because it is believed to bring blessings from the moon, it is known as the "tree of enchantment."

The History of Aspirin

The medicinal powers of willow reside within its inner bark. It is a source of salicylic acid, the active ingredient that inspired the creation of pharmaceutical aspirin. Its therapeutic abilities are well documented, and the Chinese have been familiar with willow's pain-relieving and inflammation-reducing properties since 500 BC. In the late 1750s, Rev. Edmund Stone of England used willow as a substitute for the expensive quinine bark (*Cinchona pubescens*) on his parishioners to treat fevers and chills from malaria. When the colonists came to North America, they found that the Native Americans were using willow to treat similar complaints.

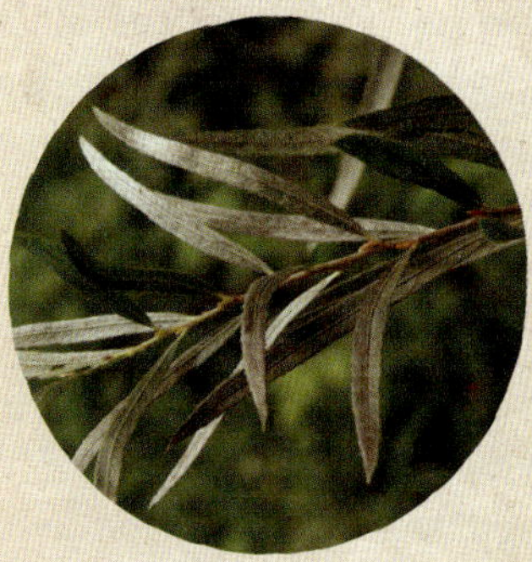

The bark provides a source of aspirin

The therapeutic compound salicin was extracted from willow bark in 1828-29 by various French and German chemists, and from this, salicylic acid was isolated in laboratories. It wasn't until Charles Gerhardt added an acetyl group to this compound in 1853 to create acetylsalicylic acid that a primitive form of aspirin was born. This research was almost forgotten until 50 years later, when a German druggist, Felix Hoffman, employed by Bayer and Company, was looking for a better rheumatoid arthritis medication for his father and read about willow's benefits in old medical journals. His father found it effectively relieved the pain, causing few side effects. Hoffman brought his findings to his superiors, and in 1899 Bayer marketed the world's first synthetic drug under the brand name Aspirin. It quickly became the remedy of choice for fever, pain and inflammation and is still one of the most widely used drugs in the world today. Due to recent studies showing aspirin's efficacy as an anti-clotting agent that helps reduce the risk of heart disease, it has made a resurgence in the marketplace.

Although salicin was first discovered in the bark of willow, it was research done on meadowsweet, *Filipendula ulmaria* (formerly *Spirea ulmaria*), 10 years later, that led to the synthesizing and manufacturing of aspirin. It was actually an extract from meadowsweet that Gerhardt used to create acetylsalicylic acid. To reflect its herbal heritage, the former generic name for meadowsweet, *Spiraea*, was immortalized in the word *aspirin*. Acetylsalicylic acid was difficult to pronounce, so they took the "A" from acetyl and "spirin" from *Spiraea*, to form the word aspirin. Although aspirin is a catchy name, it seems unfair that *Spirea* gets the glory when salicin was first discovered in willow. Furthermore, willow contains more salicylates than meadowsweet, making it a more potent healer.

Medicinal Uses

Although most medicine cabinets contain aspirin, it is surprisingly rare to find someone who knows that this drug has a past with willow bark. The salicin contained within the plant becomes salicylic acid when oxidized in the body. Salicylates have natural cooling and anodyne qualities, and they offer a wonderful combination of pain-killing, fever-reducing and anti-inflammatory benefits. The therapeutic properties of willow, while initially slower to act, continue to be effective longer than aspirin and cause fewer side effects. Generally, its natural ingredients do not irritate the stomach or thin the blood. However, willow should not be given to children under the age of 16 who have a viral infection or high fever, as it may, like aspirin, contribute to Reye's syndrome. Nicolas Culpeper noted that willow "stays the heat of lust in man and woman." At one time it was prescribed for suppressing sexual desires and was once a popular form of early birth control. The bitter, astringent bark is collected in the spring from two-to three-year-old branches and made into a tincture or dried for decoctions.

Pain and Inflammation

Because willow resides near water, folk medicine regarded it as a treatment for rheumatism, ague (a type of malarial fever often spread by mosquitos) and other illnesses aggravated by cold and damp. Due to its analgesic and anti-inflammatory properties, willow continues to be used throughout the world as a safe source of "natural aspirin." It has the ability to alleviate pain and treat inflamed conditions, such as rheumatism, arthritis, gout and swollen joints. It is an effective pain manager for sore muscles, strains, lower back aches, neuralgia, fibromyalgia and menstrual cramps, and can be useful in cases of sprains and tendonitis where the connective tissues are inflamed. The twigs have historically been chewed as a gentle pain reliever for headaches, toothaches and earaches.

Reduces Fevers

Because of willow's anti-pyretic properties, it is recommended as an effective remedy to help reduce fevers and chills associated with colds, influenza and other infections. At one time, children with a fever were bathed in a willow decoction.

Skin Care

Many early herbalists also focused on willow's antiseptic and astringent qualities for slowing bleeding and treating wounds. A bark poultice, softened by boiling, or an external wash applied to the skin not only promotes the healing of sores, ulcers, rashes, minor burns and wounds but also reduces infection.

Bach's Flower Remedies

In *Bach's Flower Remedies*, willow essence is believed to alleviate bitterness and resentment, and benefit those who blame others for their problems. It profits people who feel victimized or mistreated, and remain embittered after having suffered hardships or misfortunes. Its use inspires the healing of longstanding hurts and outstanding issues.

Other Uses

Willows are most famous for their pliable osiers or branches, which can be woven into wicker items. They were traditionally made into baskets, mats, lobster pots and bee hives, and wattle fences were once a common sight, protecting gardens and containing livestock. Today, the craft of weaving willow is enjoying a resurgence, and wicker baskets of various shapes and sizes are made using the same techniques as those in the sixth century. Also gaining popularity are landscape sculptures and outdoor seating made from live cuttings, which, due to their watery origins, are able to resist weather damage. The Indigenous people used the branches to construct racks for drying meat and fish, frames for stretching hides and framework for sweat lodges. The fibrous inner bark was twisted into cordage, twine and fishing nets. These nets were brittle when dry but strong and durable when wet and didn't soften in water like suet nets.

The wood has also been a useful friend for centuries. It is the tree of choice for making polo balls, artificial limbs, and cricket bats and wickets, due to its ability to absorb shock without splitting. It holds nails well and is durable in water, traits that are valued for manufacturing water wheels and boat keels. Being uniform in texture, lightweight and durable, it is touted as one of the traditional materials for making Dutch wooden shoes and clogs. It is also constructed into wooden crates and boxes, harvested for pulp, and commercially grown as biomass. Willow, however, makes inferior fuel wood and folklore advises not to burn it, "lest sadness befall upon you." Perhaps this superstition stemmed from the belief that the soul of the tree dies if cut for this purpose.

As late as 1826, willow twigs were used to record payment of taxes in Britain. To document the amount of taxes paid, a twig was notched and then split lengthwise. The taxpayer kept half as a receipt and the tax collector kept the other. When English tax records were converted to paper, these willow twigs were taken out and burned. Willow twigs were also made into whistles to "whistle up the wind" and were said to call in the ravens.

Tree-Top Inspiration

Weeping willow has a majestic presence in the landscape, and it is easy to appreciate how they became a muse to artists and writers. Being in the company of willow was considered to enhance your visionary skills, allowing poets, painters and musicians to gain insight, inspiration and clarity of mind. This practice was known to the Celts as "gaining tree-top inspiration," an expression still used today. It was considered that sitting with a willow tree was advantageous when starting new projects. Even now, willow continues its association with the arts, providing one of the finest drawing charcoals favoured by artists. This same charcoal, which reduces to almost pure carbon, was also manufactured into gun powder, and some black powder purists still use it, touting it as one of the best.

A Symbol of Grief

Willows were planted in gardens during the romantic era to evoke a mournful mood in the landscape, and they were commonly depicted in art, or portrayed in poetry and music as an expression of romantic melancholy. In folklore, weeping willow's drooping branches came to portray sadness and were associated with death, heartbreak, loneliness, sorrow and lost love.

Willow's connection with grief and sorrow was depicted as far back as biblical times. Psalm 137, regarding the captive Israelites, says, "By the rivers of Babylon we sat down and wept when we remembered Zion. There on the willow trees we hung up our harps." Although the willows that grew beside the river of Babylon were most likely poplars, the weeping willow still holds the botanical name *Salix babylonica* and continues to be associated with sadness.

Willows were connected with funerals, and during Medieval times sprigs of willow were worn as a sign of grief to indicate you were in mourning. They were also carried to allay the fear of death and planted near burial sites in Britain as guardian trees to protect the dead from evil influences and to ease the passage of souls into the afterlife. By the nineteenth century illustrations of weeping willows were commonly depicted on gravestones and mourning cards.

The ancient Celts also associated willow with grief and believed the flowing branches helped release sorrow and despair, and swept away the tears. Willow was able to heal the human spirit by easing sadness from lost loved ones or matters of the heart. Its nurturing love aided in the grieving process, helping a person move through their emotions to facilitate healing and allow the pain to be expressed through tears. Studies now show that dozens of biochemical components within willows that are readily released into the air and absorbed through the lungs may help with loneliness and mild depression.

Forsaken in Love

Furthermore, willow came to symbolize unrequited love or the loss of a lover. In the sixteenth and seventeenth century, grief suffered by those who had been forsaken in love or rejected by a lover for another, adopted the custom of wearing a garland or sprig of willow in their hat to indicate they were in mourning. "Willow hats" were presented to those who were disappointed in love, and expressions like "where is your willow hat", or "to wear the willow" came from this tradition and meant to grieve openly. A Greek proverb stated that men must pause to touch willow growing along water when they pass; otherwise, they would lose their sweetheart. In Medieval times the leaves were also worn as a charm to protect against jealousy.

Protection

Considered to have protective powers, willow was planted in gardens to shield homes, watch over families and guard against negative influences. It was believed that, when hung over doors, it kept "swamp witches" and other evil spirits at bay. In Mexico, when severe storms threatened, people would invoke the aid of the gods by praying to the willow tree. On Palm Sunday in Britain, crosses were made of willow and kept until the following year to protect homes and act as "thunder" charms.

Because it was considered lucky to carry on journeys, the Druids made rods from willow twigs, known as sally rods, as protective charms. A traditional verse goes as follows: "knock on willow three by three times and no evil will follow thee." An ancient custom held that evil could be averted and bad luck sent away by knocking on a willow tree; this is likely where the expression "to knock on wood" or "touch wood" originated, meaning to prevent or ward off misfortune.

Willows are not always perceived as holding protective powers. An old Somerset folksong warned travelers of the dangers of willows, telling how they would uproot themselves at night and stalk unsuspecting visitors. In J.K. Rowling's book *Harry Potter and the Chamber of Secrets*, the students at Hogwarts needed to contend with the Whomping Willow. Although this foul-tempered tree was assigned to be the guardian of the back entrance to the Shrieking Shack, its concern for the welfare of the students was not apparent, as it smacked any who came near its branches.

Folklore

Willow groves are considered magical places where meditation and visionary skills are enhanced. Being in the company of willows is believed to increase psychic and intuitive powers, providing the gift of prophecy so that dreams are more vivid and open to interpretation and understanding. Its wood is favoured for making divining rods to locate water, find lost objects and channel earth's energy. The Medieval Irish were renowned for their harp skills and claimed that willows have souls that speak through music; thus, many carved their instruments from willow wood.

There are many tales of nymphs or tree spirits livings in willows. Some venture among humans during the day but return to the willow at night. The term "wind in the willow" refers to these spirits whispering among themselves, which can be heard when walking beneath the tree.

Sometimes referred to as "hollow willow," it is believed a secret confessed to a willow is trapped in the tree forever, thus your secret is kept safe. Tying a willow twig into a knot while expressing a wish, will encourage it to come true. Leave it on a branch, and when it has been granted, return to the tree and untie the knot. Be sure to thank the tree before leaving.

The besom, or the traditional witch's broom, was customarily made from three trees, each incorporating their magical qualities. The ash handle was used for protection and enhanced one's ability to work with the four elements, the birch twigs, used for the brush, enticed helpful spirits into one's service, and the willow that bound the birch twigs to the staff connected one to the moon and the feminine energies of the goddess.

To determine whether you will marry within the year, on New Year's Eve throw your boot or shoe into a willow tree. If it gets caught in the branches within seven tries, you will wed within twelve months. A drawback with this infallible prediction is that you will need to climb the tree to retrieve your boot should it become snagged.

The Energy of Willow

Known for her unique beauty and spiritual presence, willow carries with her the energy of flowing water. She is considered to be a source of gentle humility and kindness, speaking to us with elegance and gracious love. The drooping branches form a fountain shape that bubbles up and over her sides, releasing a peaceful energy that softly spreads out from her limbs to nurture a sense of calm and tranquility beneath. People and wildlife go to her for serenity and comfort.

Lessons of the Willow

Willow can reconnect us with our intuitive side. She allows us to associate with the spirits of passed loved ones and deal with our loss by bringing sorrow to the surface and permitting us to let it go. Her essence restores optimism and faith to those feeling resentment and bitterness, and encourages the release of deeply buried feelings, sadness and pain through tears and grieving. Willow's moon energy also reminds us we need to surrender our deepest emotions to the water world so that we may overcome our fears and weaknesses.

As demonstrated by her shoots that readily sprout, willow supports growth and healing, helping us move towards a greater acceptance of self and others. Furthermore, her supple twigs teach us that sometimes we need to be more flexible, inspiring us to adapt to life changes rather than resisting. Other times we just need to go with the flow and sit on the river bank in the shade of a giant willow, watching the water gently drift by.

Witch Hazel

Hamamelis virginiana

Snapping Hazel, Snap Alder, Winter Bloom, Water Wizard, Diviner and Tobacco Wood

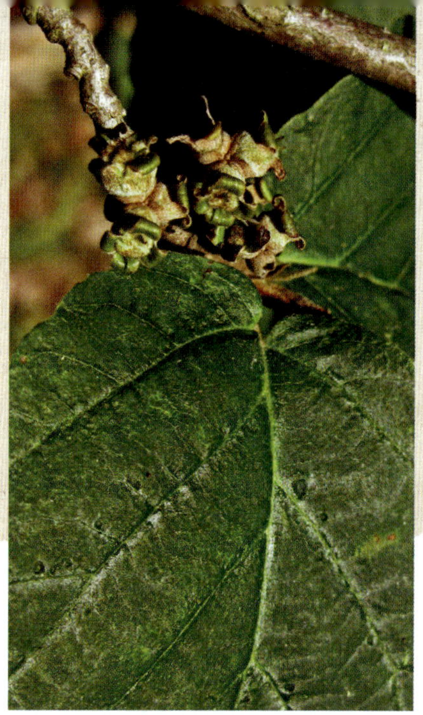

There is something almost supernatural about witch hazel, as few plants can match it for its bewitching powers. It seems appropriately named as its gnarled, misshaped stems give it a spooky appearance and the clusters of spidery-like flowers materialize at Halloween. The mysterious spitting seeds, which create a startling bang, are surely evidence of occult influences. Early colonists used its branches to make brooms, the witches' favorite mode of transportation, and they have special magical powers to divine or "witch" underground water and precious metals, once an art associated with witchcraft. It is even rumoured to have the ability to remove unwanted hexes. Clearly witch hazel makes a great candidate as a Halloween plant and the mysteries associated with it.

Meeting Witch Hazel

Slow growing and classified as either a shrub or small tree, witch hazel is usually found in the understory of deciduous forests. It tolerates both sunny and shady locations, but produces more flowers and fruit when provided with ample light. Its root sends up several sinuous, crooked stems, which together form an open, umbrella-like crown of twisted, flexible branches, and the entire plant creates a beautiful silhouette against the winter sky.

Witch hazel is an irresistible addition to gardens, providing the right mix of beauty and mystery, and because it grows only ten to fifteen feet tall it is particularly suited for small areas. A garden bench tucked

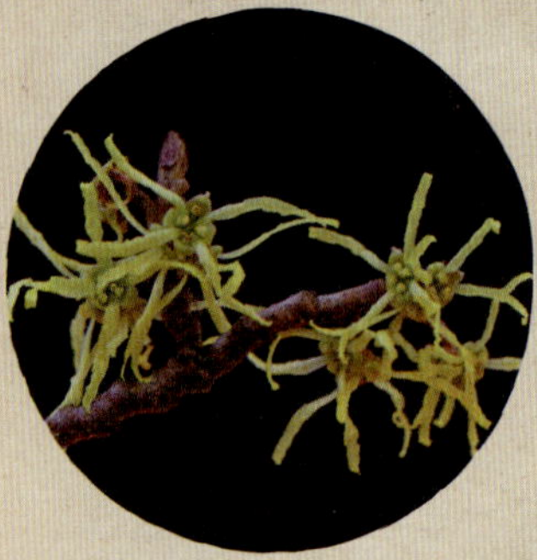

Witch hazel blooms in late fall

beneath its canopy makes a picturesque setting welcoming those strolling through to stop and rest for a while. It is native to eastern North America but over the years has received much attention and is now widely planted elsewhere. In the 1700s it was taken back to England as a garden ornamental for its ability to grow in semi-shade, its attractive, multi-stemmed shape and its unique autumn blooms. Recently, many cultivars have been developed, satisfying a variety of garden preferences.

Late Bloomers

The leaves have a wavy, scalloped margin with an uneven base and are spectacular in the fall when they display their rich, golden beauty. The strange, scraggly flowers too are very intriguing. Each has four twisted, ribbon-like petals that look like tiny golden torches cloaking the branches. However, what really makes them unique is the fact that they bloom in late fall, even after their autumn leaves have dropped, creating a nice contrast in the dormant landscape when few other plants are in flower. They appear to have their own little heartbeat, seemingly defying the wintery cold. On frosty days they curl up their petals, only to open them again when the sun comes out and warms the cold air. Due to this trait, witch hazel is sometimes known as "winter bloom."

Pollination

The fragrant flowers attract insects to aid fertilization, but because few pollinators are active so late in the season, studies have shown that insects not normally considered pollinators assist in transporting the pollen. Witch hazels are not picky which insects make use of them, and visitors such as small gnats, parasitoid wasps, noctuid moths, hover flies and tachinid flies have all been noted. Each flower can last up to a month, giving potential pollinators plenty of time to find them. Furthermore, to compensate for the fact that they bloom at a time when most insects are dormant, they have also evolved to self-pollinate if the need arises.

Although pollination takes place in autumn, actual fertilization of the ovules does not occur until spring. This practice is similar to delayed implantation common in the weasel family. The seeds then develop and mature over the summer and disperse the following fall when the new blooms appear.

Exploding Seeds

The fruit are small woody capsules that persist on the plant throughout the year. Each pod holds two hard, shiny seeds, and it takes a full year for them to ripen inside. Witch hazel has an unusual life cycle, operating on a different calendar than most plants. While the flowers are blooming, the seed pods from the previous year are opening and ejecting their black seeds. Hence, it produces flowers, drops its leaves, goes dormant, and spreads its seeds all at the same time—activities most plants spread over several months.

Another interesting phenomenon is their seed-dispersing mechanism. When the temperature and humidity are ideal, the mature seeds are violently driven from their dry capsules, creating a loud snapping sound. They are propelled with such force that they are often shot a distance of three to nine meters (ten to thirty feet) from the tree. This characteristic gave rise to the common names snapping hazel and snap alder. Once expelled, the seed commonly lies dormant on the ground two winters before germinating.

Meaning of its Name

Despite all its witchy, magical qualities, the name has no association with witches from the Medieval period; but rather "*witch*" was derived from "*wych*," an old Anglo-Saxon word related to the word *wicker* that means bendable or pliant. The name is most likely referencing its flexible twigs and twisted shape. The genus name *Hamamelis* is derived from a Greek word meaning "together with fruit," speaking of its tendency to retain last year's fruit while the new flowers are blooming.

The History of Distilled Witch Hazel

Witch hazel was a highly valued remedy used by the North American Indigenous people, whose knowledge of its medicinal properties has since been confirmed accurate. They believed it to be a gift from the Great Spirit and considered it an important ceremonial herb. When North America was being settled by European immigrants, the Indigenous people brought its medicinal virtues to their attention and it was quickly adopted. They widely used it for its ability to treat cuts, wounds, burns, bruises and hemorrhoids, and in 1860 it was listed in the *Pharmacopoeia of the United States*. However, by the middle of the nineteenth century, it was distilled witch hazel water prepared from the fresh twigs that was found in most bathroom cabinets and a much-used remedy in the days of our grandmothers and great grandmothers. It is still widely available as an over-the-counter item in most drug stores for topical use and is one of the most convenient and easy to use astringents for treating various skin conditions.

The man behind popularizing this product was Theron T. Pond, a pharmacist from Utica, New York. In the early 1840s he became friends with an Oneida healer who advocated this herb for treating wounds and burns. Together, in 1846, they prepared and patented the first commercial witch hazel preparation called Golden Treasure, which later became known as Pond's Extract. It was one of the first American mass-marketed commercial remedies, and today it is still sold under the same name as a mild astringent and antiseptic for minor abrasions and skin irritations, and as a skin toner.

Originally, early witch hazel water was simply a decoction of the plant, and due to its tannin content, it was highly astringent. This made it an excellent healing remedy when an astringent property was called for. However, by the late nineteenth century, manufacturers switched to steam distillation. Here the plant was soaked in water and the resulting infusion was distilled. Ethyl alcohol was added to keep the distillate from spoiling. This process left little of the plant's astringent tannins. *King's American Dispensatory* (1898), the textbook used by Eclectic physicians, noted that the decoction is useful for numerous ailments but stated that "since the introduction of the distilled extract, (witch hazel) has been largely abandoned ... the fluid extract has little to recommend it." *The Dispensatory of the United States* also indicated that the distilled extract had little to offer and "serves only in filling the needs in American families for ailments which appeals to the psychic influence of faith." Although there is some question of its medicinal value, it has been marketed for 175 years and more than one million gallons of bottled distilled witch hazel are sold each year in the United States. This makes it one of the most widely used healing herbs made from a wild North American plant.

So, is there any value in distilled witch hazel water? Although the distilled preparation contains

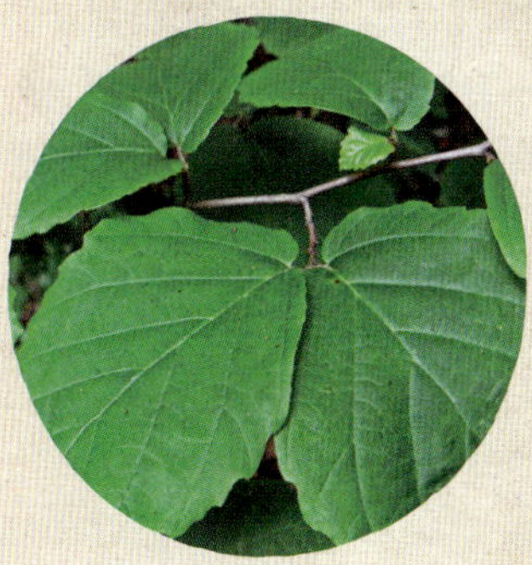

The branches are used to divine underground water sources

little of its original tannins, several studies have shown that it still upholds an astringent action, suggesting there are other astringent principles within the plant. It also has been shown to have antiseptic, anesthetic and anti-inflammatory qualities, making it useful for many of the issues it was originally promoted for, including treating burns, cuts, scrapes, bruises, acne, rashes, itching, hemorrhoids, sprains, inflammation, insect bites and stings and other minor skin conditions.

Medicinal Uses

A decoction made from the twigs and leaves has long been of service and was highly valued for centuries in North American medicine. It was listed as a mild astringent and anti-inflammatory in the *United States Pharmacopoeia* (1862 to 1916) and *National Formulary* (1861 to 1955). Distilled witch hazel water found at pharmacies is not the same as witch hazel decoction and tincture, and many herbal practitioners prefer these later preparations because it is the tannins that give this classic remedy its toning properties. Not only is witch hazel well documented for its astringent influences, it is also antiseptic and hemostatic (checks bleeding), and its cooling and drying qualities make it useful for soothing and toning varicose veins, hemorrhoids, bruises, swellings and other skin problems. As well, it may exhibit antiviral activities, being used with great advantage against the herpes simplex virus.

It is the bark and sometimes the leaves that are utilized. Harvest the branches in spring and strip off the inner bark to make a decoction or low-alcohol tincture (25% alcohol). The leaves are gathered throughout summer and dried quickly in a shady location. Both are used to create washes, ointments, salves, douches and other external preparations whenever an astringent remedy is required. It is quite safe for topical use; however, due to its strong astringent action, some herbalists advise against taking internally.

Hemorrhoids

Witch hazel's soothing and toning properties are particularly ideal for shrinking and easing hemorrhoids, and it is commonly found in commercial preparations for this purpose. It has the ability to strengthen the veins and improve debilitated circulation; therefore, it is specific for hemorrhoids caused by a weakened circulatory system that lacks tone. When applied externally as a cooling compress, ointment, or sitz bath, it effectively reduces swelling, bleeding and pain.

Varicose Veins

This healing astringent has a special influence upon the venous circulation and is particularly useful for varicose veins. This disease arises when the veins become distended and distorted from loss of elasticity and can make walking and sitting very uncomfortable. When applied externally, witch hazel's constricting action on the vascular walls helps to tighten and tone enlarged veins and provide relief from pain and discomfort. Witch hazel also supports other diseases characterized by venous dilatation or relaxation causing feeble circulation, which in turn can burden the kidneys and heart and result in conditions such as edema.

Cuts and Wounds

The tannins in witch hazel aid in wound healing by slowing bleeding, reducing swelling and providing antiseptic actions. A compress helps mend and clean cuts and abrasions by drawing the skin together and discouraging infection; and its cooling, astringent action makes it effectual in reducing inflammation and staunching minor bleeding. Inflamed and irritated skin responds well to witch hazel, making this herb ideal for a variety of complaints. It is advantageous for relieving itchy rashes, poison ivy, psoriasis, eczema, insect bites, stings, minor burns and sunburns, and is an herbal ally for slow-healing ulcers, old sores and painful tumors. It is also a classic treatment for bruises and is often combined with arnica, yarrow and St John's wort for this purpose.

Musculoskeletal Issues

Furthermore, its anti-inflammatory and pain-relieving properties benefit the swelling and discomfort from sprains, strains, back pain, arthritic joints and achy muscles. A decoction or tincture was also rubbed on legs of athletes to keep them limber.

Eyes, Mouth and Gums

A compress is very efficacious in alleviating red, puffy eyes and benefits all manners of soreness, infection or inflammation. It is excellent for ruptured blood vessels in the eye or a blow to the eye causing swelling and bruising.

Witch hazel's virtues also make it a major herbal ally for oral issues and an excellent choice for bleeding gums and inflamed mouth sores. A mouth wash helps heal infections, strengthen the gums and tighten the teeth. Use a strong tea or put a few drops of witch hazel tincture on a wet toothbrush and gently brush along the gum line.

Cosmetic Uses

Distilled witch hazel extract is commonly found in hair rinses, soaps and skin care products, as well as commercial aftershave lotions and mouthwashes. This essential beauty aid is regularly added to cosmetic and first aid products for its light astringent, toning and cleansing gifts and is particularly useful for puffiness around the eyes and to heal spider veins. Its mild antibacterial properties are valued as a cleanser in treating pimples, acne and other skin blemishes, and a cotton pad soaked in the distilled water removes makeup, tightens the pores and gently cleans the skin, giving it a tingling sensation. As well, it is widely used as a rinse for oily hair and skin, and benefits liver or sun spots. Be sure to use the distilled water as a daily facial toner because the decoction can become too astringent and drying.

Water Witching

One of witch hazel's gifts is its ability to locate underground water sources. The forked branches were traditionally employed by both Native Americans and colonists as divining rods to "witch water." The wood was also said to afford special powers in pointing to concealed salt, gold, silver and other precious metals. Old-timers have even found lost household items, tools, knives and old grave sites in abandoned cemeteries. This ancient method for finding or chasing water and other objects provided witch hazel with other common names such as "water wizard" or "diviner."

My father had an art for dowsing water. He would cut a living Y-shaped branch from the witch hazel and take a prong in each hand. While holding the branch in front of him parallel with the ground, he gripped each prong loosely in his hands with his palms up and thumbs pointing out and away from his body. At this point, he would slowly start to walk back and forth. When a large accumulation of underground water was detected, the "witch stick" would generate a bobbing action or the main stem would turn towards the ground, indicating the location of the hidden stream.

Folklore

Witch hazel was believed to have the ability to banish unwanted emotions and remove hexes, diseases and general negativity. Additionally, if carried, it was thought to help mend a broken heart. It could heighten the power of prayers, charms or spells, launching them in the right direction, and a wand waved over a road, path or stream could determine if good or evil had passed that way. In the Ozark Hills, the twigs were tied into equal-arm crosses and hung on barns to safeguard their animals and encourage benevolent spirits.

Perhaps because of its affinity to finding water, it was used in weather magic. An old cure for warts was to cut three notches in a witch hazel twig and cast it into a running stream.

Lessons of Witch Hazel

Just as witch hazel has the ability to find water, it has an uncanny knack for revealing the truth. When placed in meetings, it ensures an honest discussion and allows people to share their feelings without reservation or fear of consequences. Furthermore, it is capable of finding optimistic energy to clear the way for a positive outcome. Because it blooms out of season, the flower essence can be used when your life is feeling out of sync. Like willow, the pliant branches also remind us to be flexible and teach us to bend when the need arises.

References

Bennett, Robin Rose. The Gift of Healing Herbs. North Atlantic Books, Berkeley, California, 2014

Beresford-Kroeger, Diana. Arboretum America: A Philosophy of the Forest. The University of Michigan Press, Ann Arbor, Michigan, 2003

Beresford-Kroeger, Diana. Arboretum Borealis: A Lifeline of the Planet. The University of Michigan Press, Ann Arbor, Michigan, 2010

Bouchardon, Patrice. The Healing Energies of Trees. Journey Editions, Boston, Massachusetts, 1999

Brown, Tom, Jr. Wild Edible and Medicinal Plants. Berkley Books, New York, New York, 1985

Bruton-Seal, Julie and Matthew Seal. Backyard Medicine. Skyhorse Publishing, New York, New York, 2009

Castleman, Michael. The New Healing Herbs. Rodale Inc., United States, 2009

Cunningham, Scott. Encyclopedia of Magical Herbs. Llewellyn Publications, St. Paul's, Minnesota, 1995

Eastman, John. The Book of Forest and Thicket. Stackpole Books, Harrisburg, Pennsylvania, 1992

Eastman, John. The Book of Swamp and Bog. Stackpole Books, Mechanicsburg, Pennsylvania, 1995

Erichsen-Brown, Charlotte. Use of Plants for the Last 500 Years. Breezy Creeks Press, Aurora, Ontario, 1979

Foster, Steven and Rebecca Johnson. Desk Reference to Nature's Medicine. National Geographic, Washington D.C., 2006

Gifford, Jane. The Wisdom of Trees. Godsfield Press, Great Britain, 2000

Gladstar, Rosemary. Family Herbal. Storey Books, North Adams, Massachusetts, 2001

Green, James. The Herbal Medicine-Makers Handbook. Crossing Press, Berkeley, California, 2000

Grieve, Mrs. Maude. A Modern Herbal. 1931. Two Volumes. Dover Publications, Inc., New York, New York, 1971

Griggs, Barbara. The Green Witch:

A Modern Women's Herbal. Random House, London, England, 1993
Groves, Maria Noel. Body into Balance. Storey Books, North Adams, Massachusetts, 2016
Hoffmann, David. The New Holistic Herbal. Element Book Limited, Shaftesbury, Dorset, 1983 and 1990
Hopman, Ellen Evert. A Druid's Herbal; For the Sacred Earth Year. Destiny Books, Rochester, Vermont, 1995
Hutchens, Alma R. Indian Herbalogy of North America. Merco, Windsor, Ontario, 1969
Kloss, Jethro. Back to Eden. 1939
MacKinnon, Kershaw, Arnason, Owen, Karst, Hamersley and Chambers. Edible and Medicinal Plants of Canada. Lone Pine Publishing, Edmonton, Alberta, 2009
Marieb, Elaine. Essentials of Human Anatomy and Physiology. Ninth Edition. Pearson Benjamin Cummings, San Francisco, California, 2009
Mills, Simon. Out of the Earth. Viking Arkana, London, England, 1991
Peterson, Lee. A Field Guide to Edible Wild Plants of Eastern and Central North America. Houghton Mifflin Company, Boston, Massachusetts, 1978
Rupp, Rebecca. Red Oaks and Black Birches. Storey Communications, Inc., Pownal, Vermont, 1994
Stuart, Malcolm. The Encyclopedia of Herbs and Herbalism. Orbis Publishing, London, England, 1979
Tallamy, Douglas W. Bringing Nature Home. Timber Press, Portland, Oregon, 2009
Vickery, Roy. Oxford Dictionary of Plant-Lore. Oxford University Press, England, 1995
Wohlleben, Peter. The Hidden Life of Trees. Greystone Books, Vancouver, British Columbia and Berkeley, California, 2015
Wood, Matthew. The Book of Herbal Wisdom. North Atlantic Books, Berkeley, California, 1977
Wood, Matthew. The Earthwise Herbal: A Complete Guide to Old World Medicinal Plants. North Atlantic Books, Berkeley, California, 2008
Wood, Matthew. The Earthwise Herbal: A Complete Guide to New World Medicinal Plants. North Atlantic Books, Berkeley, California, 2009

RELATED TITLES

View all Hancock House titles at hancockhouse.com

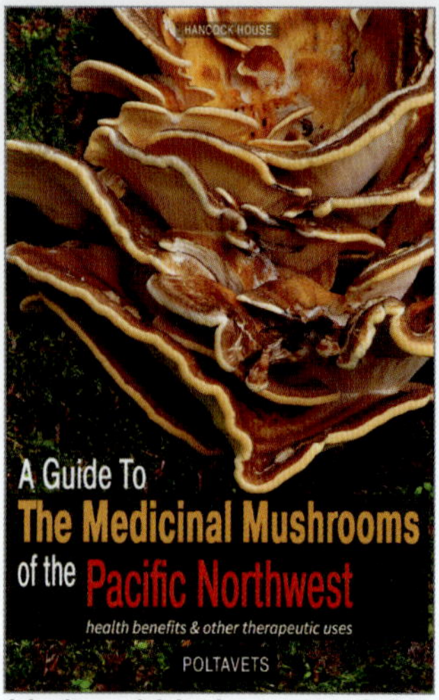

Medicinal Mushrooms of the PNW
Svetlana Poltavets
ISBN 9780888393517 SC
$14.95

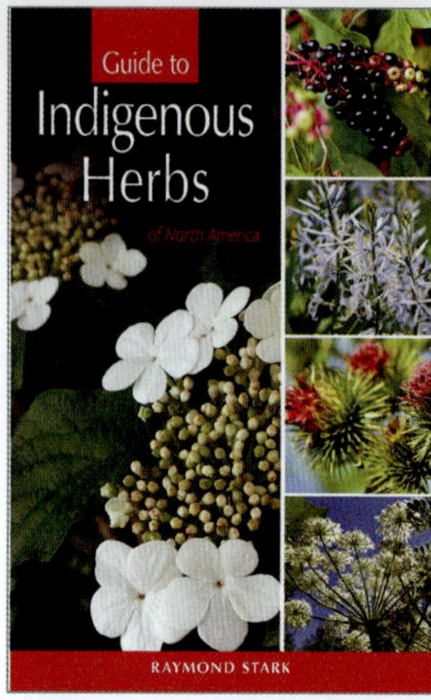

Indigenous Herbs
Ray Stark
ISBN 9780888390776 SC
$11.95

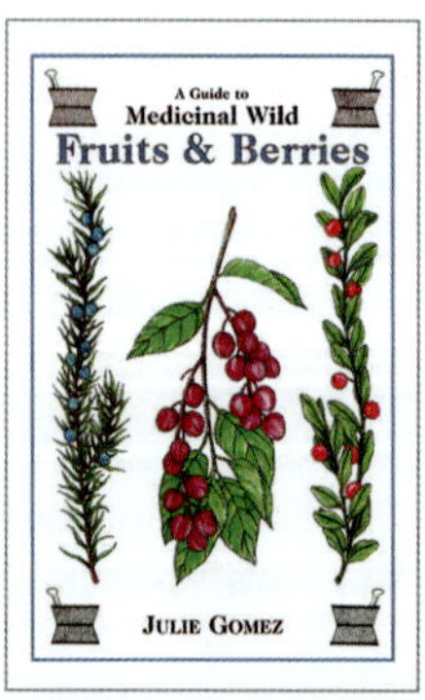

Medicinal Wild Fruits and Berries
Julie Gomez
ISBN 9780888394453 SC

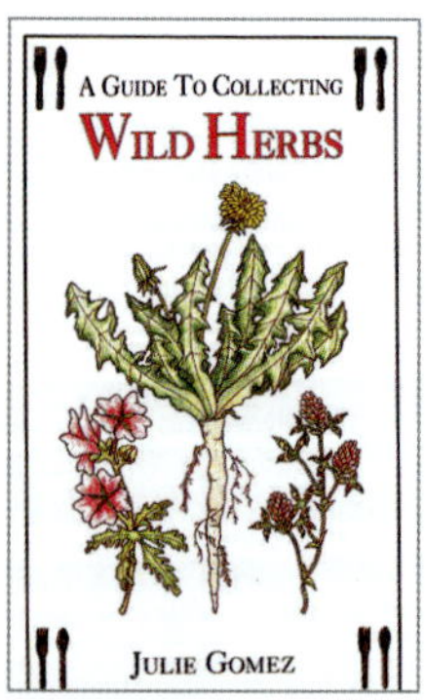

Wild Herbs
Julie Gomez
ISBN 9780888393975 SC

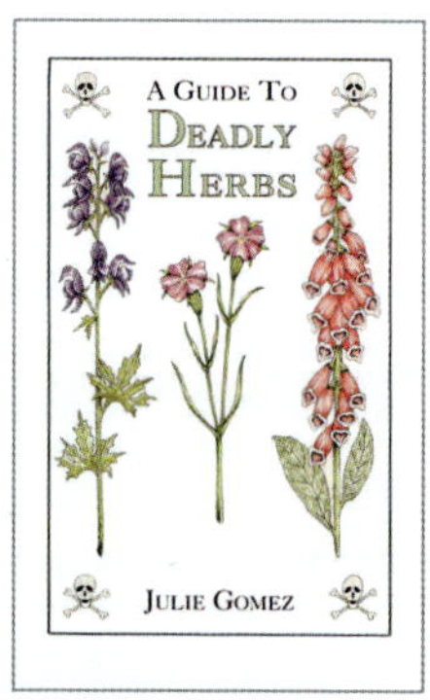

Deadly Herbs
Julie Gomez
ISBN 9780888393906 SC

Hancock House Publishers
19313 Zero Ave, Surrey, BC
V3Z 9R9
www.hancockhouse.com
info@hancockhouse.com
1-800-938-1114

From an early age, Brenda Gallagher was captivated by the beauty and mystery of the natural world—a fascination nurtured by her parents and grandparents, who introduced her to its wonders. Over the past 35 years, she has cultivated a deep passion for medicinal plants, studying their uses and sharing her knowledge through presentations, workshops, and interpretive hikes. An avid gardener and forager, she delights in growing and gathering herbs to craft her own healing remedies. Brenda currently serves as a vegetation specialist with the Upper Thames River Conservation Authority in Southern Ontario, where she leads natural restoration projects that help heal and protect the land she loves.

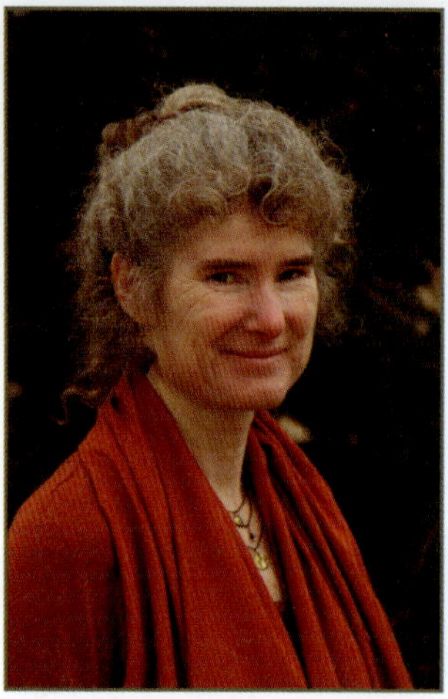